A clinician's brief guide to children's mental health law

Sarah Huline-Dickens

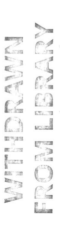

RCPsych Publications

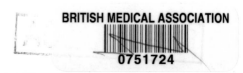

RCPsych Publications is an imprint of the Royal College of Psychiatrists,
21 Prescot Street, London E1 8BB
http://www.rcpsych.ac.uk

British Library Cataloguing-in-Publication Data.
A catalogue record for this book is available from the British Library.
ISBN 978-1-909726-71-0

Distributed in North America by Publishers Storage and Shipping Company.

The views presented in this book do not necessarily reflect those of the Royal
College of Psychiatrists, and the publishers are not responsible for any error of
omission or fact.

The Royal College of Psychiatrists is a charity registered in England and Wales
(228636) and in Scotland (SC038369).

Contains public sector information licensed under the Open Government
Licence v3.0.

Printed by Bell & Bain Limited, Glasgow, UK

Contents

Foreword

Interdisciplinarity has long been recognised as a vital component of the family justice system and also, one hopes, of the criminal justice system. In the family justice system, though seemingly not in the criminal justice system, interdisciplinarity has come of age, with the increasing recognition of the need to rebalance the system through a much greater use of problem-solving courts. Psychiatrists and other professionals will no longer feature just as expert witnesses, helping the judge to establish what has happened and to craft some kind of solution; they will be key parts of an interdisciplinary team, including but not limited to the judge, seeking to understand, to address and to resolve the underlying problems.

There is, however, a difficulty. Any justice system of its very nature applies the law and operates in accordance with processes devised by lawyers and expressed in legalese. And, as our author tactfully reminds us with her very apposite reference to Dickens's Mr Kenge, lawyers are not always very good at explaining to non-lawyers what the law is or how the legal system operates. That is why we need practitioners' handbooks, whether for the use, for example, of social workers or, as here, for the use of psychiatrists, written by experienced practitioners in the relevant discipline who understand better than lawyers what their fellow practitioners need and how best to present it in a way which meets those needs.

That is why this excellent handbook, written by a distinguished and forensically experienced consultant in child and adolescent psychiatry, is so important and why it will, I am sure, be so valuable. Ultimately, the judges of Dr Sarah Huline-Dickens's success in writing this handbook will be her professional colleagues. As a mere lawyer, all I can say is that it deserves every success and that it will, I expect, be of very great assistance to those in her professional community who need a reliable and accessible guide to what may be unfamiliar when their work takes them into the forensic context. I wish it well.

James Munby
President of the Family Division
2 September 2016

Acknowledgements

I would like to thank the following:

Mr Justice Baker

Dr Michael Carter

Elizabeth Evans

Dr Stephen Goss

Jeffrey Hackney

Sir James Munby

Janice Parker-Elliott

Dr Andy Sant

Lee Snook

List of cases

If the year of publication is essential to identifying the case it is written in square brackets [ ]. If the date is ancillary it is in rounded brackets ( ).

A Local Authority v A (a child) & Anor [2010] EWHC 978.

AM v South London & Maudsley NHS Foundation Trust [2013] UKUT 365 (AAC).

An NHS Trust v A [2015] EWCOP 71.

Birmingham City Council v Riaz & Ors (Rev 2) [2014] EWHC 4247 (Fam).

Bolam v Friern Hospital Management Committee [1957] WLR 582.

Gillick v West Norfolk and Wisbech Area Health Authority [1985] UKHL 7 (17 October 1985).

GJ v The Foundation Trust & Ors [2009] EWHC 2972 (Fam).

Guzzardi v Italy 7367/76 (1980) ECHR 5.

Herczegfalvy v Austria (1992) 15 EHRR 43.

HL v UK (2004) 40 EHRR 761.

John (M) [2003] EWCA Crim 3452.

Montgomery (Appellant) v Lanarkshire Health Board (Respondent) (Scotland) [2015] UKSC 11.

MS v UK (2012) 55 EHRR 23.

Neilsen v Denmark (1988) 11 EHRR 175.

P v Cheshire West & Chester Council and another and P and Q v Surrey County Council [2014] AC 896.

R (on the application of Axon) v Secretary of State for Health [2006] EWHC 37 (Admin).

R (on the application of B) v Stafford Combined Court [2006] EWHC 1645 (admin).

R (on the application of H) v Mental Health Review Tribunal, North & East London Region & Anor [2001] EWCA Civ 415.

R (on the application of N) v M & Ors [2002] EWCA Civ 1789.

R (on the application of Stevens) v Plymouth City Council & Anor [2002] EWCA Civ 388.

R (ZN) v South west London & St George's Mental Health NHS Trust (2009) CO/9457.

R v Delaney (1988) 88 Crim App Rep 33.

R v Northampton Juvenile Court, ex p Hammersmith and Fulham LBC [1985] FLR 192.

Rabone & Anor v Pennine Care NHS Foundation [2012] UKSC 2.

Re A [2010] EWHC 978 (Fam).

Re AB [2015] EWCOP 31.

Re C (A Minor) (Wardship: Medical Treatment) (No. 2) [1990] FAM 39.

Re C (Detention: Medical Treatment) [1997] 2 FLR 180.

Re C (refusal of treatment) [1994] 1 FLR 31.

Re D (A Child: Deprivation of liberty) [2015] EWHC 922 (Fam).

Re E (a minor) (medical treatment) [1991] 7 BMLR: 117–119.

Re K (Secure accommodation order: right to liberty) [2001] 2 WLR 1141.

Re MB (Medical treatment) [1997] 2 FLR 426.

Re R (A Minor) (Wardship: Medical Treatment) [1991] 3 WLR 592.

Re Roddy (a child) (identification: restriction on publication) Torbay Borough Council v News Group Newspapers [2004] All ER (D) 150 (Feb).

Re W (a minor) (medical treatment) [1992] 4 All ER 627.

Re X (Emergency Protection Orders) [2006] EWHC 510 (Fam).

Re X & Ors (Deprivation of Liberty) [2014] EWCOP 25.

RK (by her litigation friend, the Official Solicitor) v BCC & Ors [2011] EWCA Civ 1305.

Savage v South Essex Partnership NHS Foundation Trust [2008] UKHL 74.

Savage v South Essex Partnership NHS Foundation Trust [2010] EWHC 865 (QB).

Surrey County Council v P, Cheshire West and Chester Council v P [2014] UKSC 19 [2014] AC 896.

T v United Kingdom (Application 24724/94) [2000] 2 All ER 1024, [2000] Crim LR 187.

Winterwerp v The Netherlands (1979) 2 EHRR 387.

X Council v B (Emergency Protection Orders) [2004] EWHC 2015 (Fam); [2005] 1 FLR 341.

Common abbreviations and terms

AC	Approved clinician
AMHP	Approved mental health professional
BMA	British Medical Association
CAMHS	Child and adolescent mental health services
CAO	Child arrangements order
COP	Court of Protection
CPS	Crown Prosecution Service
CQC	Care Quality Commission
CTO	Community treatment order
DoH	Department of Health
DoLS	Deprivation of Liberty Safeguards
EHCP	Education, health and care plan
ECHR	European Convention on Human Rights
ECT	Electroconvulsive therapy
ECtHR	European Court of Human Rights
GMC	General Medical Council
HRA	Human Rights Act
HSCIC	Health and Social Care Information Centre
LAPSO	Legal Aid Sentencing and Punishment of Offenders Act
MCA	Mental Capacity Act
MHA	Mental Health Act
MHAC	Mental Health Act Commission
MHMDS	Mental health minimum dataset
MHT	Mental health tribunal

NR	Nearest relative
PACE	Police and Criminal Evidence Act
RC	Responsible clinician
RMO	Registered medical officer
SOAD	Second opinion appointed doctor
UNCRC	United Nations Convention on the Rights of the Child
UNICEF	United Nations International Children's Emergency Fund
YOT	Youth offending team

Law reports

AC	Appeal cases
All ER	All England reports
BMLR	Butterworths Medical Law Reports
Crim App Rep	Criminal Appeal Reports
ECHR	European Court of Human Rights
EHRR	European Human Rights Reports
EWCA	England and Wales Court of Appeal
EWCOP	England and Wales Court of Protection
EWHC	England and Wales High Court
FLR	Family Law Reports
MHLO	Mental Health Law Online
UKSC	United Kingdom Supreme Court
WLR	Weekly Law Reports

CHAPTER 1

Introducing child mental health and the law

With the increasing complexity of culture and society comes confusion. Several changes in UK legislation affecting children's mental health have taken place over the past two decades. These have included the Human Rights Act 1998 (HRA) and the case law deriving from it, the Mental Capacity Act 2005 (MCA) and, in 2007, the amendments to Mental Health Act 1983 (MHA). We therefore find ourselves in some difficulty concerning the clarity of what can and cannot be done to look after young people's mental disorders and safeguard their rights.

Fortunately, there are already good guides written specifically for clinicians on both the MHA and the MCA: *A Clinician's Brief Guide to the Mental Health Act* (Zigmond & Brindle, 2016) and *A Clinician's Brief Guide to the Mental Capacity Act* (Brindle *et al*, 2015). These cover a lot of ground, and Zigmond & Brindle's book includes how to become section 12 approved and the process of tribunals and making appeals. Neither, however, was intended to deal with the particular problems of the law as it relates to children and adolescents with mental disorders. Complementing these volumes, this book will focus on the rather peculiar relationship between a young person with a mental health disorder and the law, as mediated by family, community and doctors.

The last book published by the Royal College of Psychiatrists on child psychiatry and the law (Black *et al*, 1998) has a good deal of information about assessing parenting capacity and how to act as an expert witness, but it now seems curious that it mentions the MHA only in passing. This must indicate some quite significant shifts in the preoccupations of the specialty of child and adolescent psychiatry and its scope of practice.

In this book I will not cover court work or how to act as a witness. I will instead focus on essential elements of children's mental health law. For clinicians acting as expert witnesses many guides are available, such as *Expert Psychiatric Evidence* (Rix, 2011), which has a chapter dedicated to reports for family proceedings relating to children. Richardson & Casswell (2010) also provide useful advice. Clinicians acting as expert witnesses need to be aware of regulations in the new Children and Families Act 2014 (Part 2, section 13). It seems from recent case law that a more rigorous approach is being adopted by the courts (Hirst, 2015), and it is likely that quality standards for expert witnesses will be developed in the future.

So what does a clinician working in child and adolescent mental health services (CAMHS) need to know about the law? The new Code of Practice for the MHA begins:

> 'In addition to the Act, those responsible for the care of children and young people in hospital should be familiar with other relevant legislation, including the Children Acts 1989 and 2004, the MCA and the HRA [Human Rights Act]. They should also be aware of the United Nations Convention on the Rights of the Child (UNCRC), and keep up-to-date with relevant case law and guidance' (Department of Health, 2015: para. 19.4).

These demands are quite considerable, and the current book is intended to help by bringing all of this information together. The final section of this chapter ('Notes on individual chapters') provides a synopsis of topics covered.

Summary of major developments

Since 1998 a great deal has changed in the medico-legal landscape of children's mental health. The Care Quality Commission (CQC) assumed responsibility for monitoring the MHA in England and Wales in 2009. The preoccupation with failings in child protection has led to the issuing of a new *Working Together to Safeguard Children* booklet (HM Government, 2015a) only 2 years after the previous one. The Supreme Court has taken over the judiciary functions of the House of Lords, and a landmark case in the Supreme Court in 2015 (*Montgomery (Appellant) v Lanarkshire Health Board (Respondent) (Scotland)* [2015]) has widely been interpreted as ending the principle of the Bolam test (see p. 39) which had been established in 1957.

Case law has continued to evolve concerning the deprivation of liberty, culminating in the so-called Cheshire West case. In fact, this judgment was given on the combined cases of Cheshire West and P and Q (*P v Cheshire West & Chester Council and another and P and Q v Surrey County Council* [2014]). Some aspects of the case are relevant to adolescents, as P and Q (also known as MIG and MEG), were aged 16 and 15 at the start of the proceedings, but 18 by the time of the final hearing in 2010. Therefore, this judgment is being viewed carefully for applicability to this age group. The judgment, delivered by Lady Hale, clarified that the definition of deprivation of liberty meant that a person is 'under continuous supervision and control and [...] not free to leave'. Moreover, 'what it means to be deprived of liberty must be the same for everyone, whether or not they have physical or mental disabilities' (para. 46).

But what are the implications of this case for children and young people? When a clinician is considering admission to hospital for a reluctant young person this is an important question and is causing much concern. Before

Cheshire West, a deprivation of liberty was considered to involve three components deriving from European law: an objective element, i.e. actual confinement for a non-negligible period of time; a subjective element, i.e. that valid consent to the confinement had not been given; and that the State was responsible for the deprivation of liberty. Case law had established that although someone with parental responsibility could authorise restrictions on the liberty of their child, these could not amount to deprivation of liberty (see *RK (by her litigation friend, the Official Solicitor) v BCC & Ors* [2011].

In the case of P and Q, the conclusion was that they had both been deprived of their liberty and that the deprivation was the responsibility of the State. At paragraph 54 of the judgment, Lady Hale says that similar constraints would not necessarily amount to a deprivation of liberty 'if imposed by parents in the exercise of their ordinary parental responsibilities'. This point was picked up by Lord Neuberger at paragraph 72, in making the case that Article 5 of the Human Rights Act (that is, the right to liberty and security of person – see Chapter 2) would not normally be engaged in the situation of children living at home. However, albeit in a not very strong statement, he doubts that this would include those living with foster parents.

Thus, a deprivation of liberty applies only when the State or its agents (e.g. foster carers) are involved: not parents or adoptive parents.

The new criteria for the deprivation of liberty are that the person lacks the capacity to consent to their care/treatment arrangements; that they are under continuous supervision and control; and that are not free to leave. These elements together have been called the acid test for the deprivation of liberty, and this finding has clearly exercised all concerned and caused widespread and costly chaos. One renegade judge has ignored it, the Law Society (2015a) has issued guidelines about what constitutes a deprivation of liberty, and the Law Commission is currently processing the results of a consultation exercise which seems likely to form the outline of a new parliamentary Bill. As part of this project (Law Commission, 2015), it is possible that there will be a proposal to extend the MHA to enable treatment of mental disorders to proceed that involve a deprivation of liberty. There is also a possibility that the new system proposed to replace the Deprivation of Liberty Safeguards – called protective care – would extend to 16- and 17-year-olds.

Cases of adolescent refusal of treatment also continue to vex both clinicians and the courts in the face of mounting recognition of adolescent autonomy. Similarly, for some time now the emphasis has been shifting away from parental rights towards parental responsibility.

On a larger canvas, at the time of writing, the future of the Human Rights Act 1998 has been brought into question by the UK government. Debates in both the House of Commons and the House of Lords have occurred, with the former Prime Minister David Cameron (a Conservative) expressing interest in a British Bill of Rights. It is not known yet what this will mean for the Human Rights Act, which was introduced by the previous Labour government.

More familiarly to psychiatrists by now, there have been the changes to the MHA, which was amended in 2007, with a new Code of Practice issued in 2015 (Department of Health, 2015). The amendments to the Act have included changes to terminology, roles and aspects of treatment. For example, the definition of mental disorder has changed, and there is now a requirement in some sections for appropriate medical treatment to be available. There is the introduction of approved clinicians, responsible clinicians and approved mental health professionals. There are also some specific changes to aspects of treatment that affect individuals under 18 years of age, such as the requirement for age-appropriate environments and rules governing the administering of electroconvulsive therapy.

And finally, there have been recent changes to family law, and I highlight some of these in the next section.

The state of mental health services and the role of the CQC

The most recent report of the CQC (Care Quality Commission, 2015) on the MHA marks 5 years since this body took over the monitoring function from the Mental Health Act Commission in England. In it, attention is drawn to the fact that there is insufficient provision of tier 3 and 4 services in CAMHS and that provision and access to CAMHS are not good enough. As I will discuss in Chapter 6, there do not appear to be systems in place yet for collecting data on the number of young people detained under the MHA. The CQC has been much more concerned about the admission of children and young people to adult wards. Consequently, its system of monitoring is restricted only to young people admitted to adult wards for more than 48 hours: even admissions to such wards for less than this period are not counted.

For the adult population in England, the total number of patients detained under the MHA at the end of March 2014 was 23 531, an increase of 6% on the previous year; and the number of available beds had reduced by 8% since 2010–2011 (Care Quality Commission, 2015).

For the CAMHS clinician in many parts of the country the main concern is the lack of available beds for young people who need emergency admissions. Even if a young person can be admitted to a paediatric ward in a crisis there can be lengthy delays before a suitable tier 4 bed can be found in an adolescent unit, and then this is often far from home.

A large change to the organisation of services was brought about with the Health and Social Care Act 2012, discussed by Zigmond & Brindle (2016: p. v). This is a complex piece of legislation concerning the decentralisation of the National Health Service in England and the introduction of commissioning boards and clinical commissioning groups. This, however, need not concern us here.

The structure of the court system in England and Wales prior to 2014

The structure of the court system in England and Wales has always been rather complicated and it changed considerably in 2014.

Prior to 2014, magistrates' courts could deal with family proceedings and could make some court orders under the Children Act 1989. County courts dealt with a wider range of court orders and complex cases from the magistrates' courts. Beyond this, the family division of the High Court would hear appeals from the magistrates' court, adoption cases, wardship cases and cases involving inherent jurisdiction. The Court of Appeal was next in the hierarchy and finally the House of Lords. Thereafter, cases might go to the European Court of Justice, based in Luxembourg. A simplified structure is shown in Fig. 1.1).

The principle of judicial precedent means that every court is bound to follow decisions in the court above it in the hierarchy and courts of appeal are bound to their own past decisions. Not all cases are reported publicly.

The structure of the court system in England and Wales after 2014

The Crime and Courts Act 2013 has created a new single family court in England and Wales. Before April 2014, family cases were dealt with at family proceedings courts (which were part of the magistrates' courts), at county courts or in the family division of the High Court. Since April 2014, all family cases are dealt with in the single family court.

Magistrates' courts and the new single county court are no longer able to deal with family proceedings, and family proceedings courts have ceased to exist.

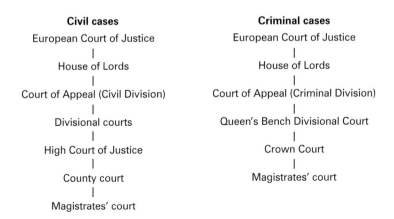

Civil cases

European Court of Justice
|
House of Lords
|
Court of Appeal (Civil Division)
|
Divisional courts
|
High Court of Justice
|
County court
|
Magistrates' court

Criminal cases

European Court of Justice
|
House of Lords
|
Court of Appeal (Criminal Division)
|
Queen's Bench Divisional Court
|
Crown Court
|
Magistrates' court

Fig. 1.1 The hierarchy of courts in England and Wales before 2014 (after Martin, 2005).

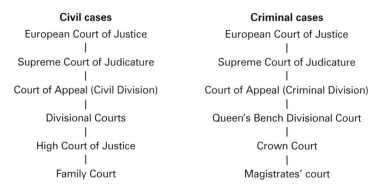

Civil cases	Criminal cases
European Court of Justice	European Court of Justice
|	|
Supreme Court of Judicature	Supreme Court of Judicature
|	|
Court of Appeal (Civil Division)	Court of Appeal (Criminal Division)
|	|
Divisional Courts	Queen's Bench Divisional Court
|	|
High Court of Justice	Crown Court
|	|
Family Court	Magistrates' court

Fig. 1.2 The hierarchy of courts in England and Wales after 2014 (adapted from Courts and Tribunals Judiciary, 2012).

However, as the family court can sit anywhere in England and Wales, in practice hearings will tend to be held in county or magistrates' court buildings.

The new family courts deal with parental disputes, local authority intervention to protect children, and domestic violence remedies and adoption. They also handle divorce petitions, and the financial provisions for children after divorce or relationship breakdown.

The judicial functions of the House of Lords were taken over by the Supreme Court in October 2009 (Fig. 1.2). The nature of the proceedings determines the court in which they are heard.

It might be helpful at this point to give some definitions. Common law refers to law that has been developed by the cumulative body of judicial decisions, i.e. by cases that have been heard in the courts. The principles thus derived are then applied to future cases, unless the new material can be legally distinguished from what has gone before. Common law is trumped by statute law, which refers to laws made by a legislative body, i.e. Acts of Parliament. Common law should not be used when there is a statutory alternative. It is also helpful to know that private law concerns relationships between private individuals, and public law is about relationships between individuals and the State.

The state of the family justice system

Statistics from the Ministry of Justice (2015*a*) indicate that, of the 60 902 cases starting in the family courts in England and Wales in January to March 2015, nearly half were divorce cases.

Since 2012, there has been a general upwards trend in the number of applications for non-molestation domestic violence protection orders and in the number of adoption orders issued.

In terms of public law orders (essentially those concerning child protection and including care or supervision orders and emergency protection orders), the most common types of order applied for in January to March 2015 were care orders (72% of children involved in applications), followed by emergency protection orders (6%) and discharge of care orders (6%).

The average time for the disposal of a care or supervision application made in January to March 2015 was 29 weeks.

The number of private law cases (largely cases under section 8 of the Children Act) started in January to March 2015 in England and Wales was 10 569 (Ministry of Justice, 2015a).

Since April 2013, legal aid has been available for private family law cases (such as those involving contact or divorce) only if there is evidence of domestic violence or child abuse and for child abduction cases. These changes are causing popular concern, as such evidence, especially of domestic violence, can be hard to produce. Legal aid remains available for public family law cases (such as adoption).

Other changes in the family justice system are reviewed in the document *A Brighter Future for Family Justice*, issued jointly by the Ministry of Justice and Department for Education (2014). This document indicates that between January 2011 and March 2014, cases concerning section 8 private law orders took on average 15–20 weeks from application to first full order.

The Crime and Security Act 2010 introduced two measures to protect victims in the immediate aftermath of the reporting of a domestic violence incident: domestic violence protection notices (DVPNs) and domestic violence protection orders (DVPOs). Police forces have been implementing these new powers since March 2014.

If the perpetrator and the victim live together, the DVPN or DVPO can exclude the perpetrator from the home or from coming within a specified distance of the home. These are temporary measures to allow time for other measures, such as applying for a civil injunction, to be taken (Ministry of Justice, 2015a).

The Children and Families Act 2014 introduced several new requirements and procedures. These include the new child arrangements orders (CAOs), which replace contact and residence orders (see Chapter 3); a 26-week time limit for completing care and supervision cases; and restricting the use of expert evidence (Law Society, 2015a). The Act also includes provisions for adoption and contact, introduces new controls over the expert witness and describes the new education, health and care plans (EHCPs). Finally, it has introduced a clause into the Children Act 1989 that encourages the court to presume, unless the contrary is shown, that involvement of each parent in the life of the child will benefit the child's welfare.

The scope of the book

In this book, I use the word 'children' to describe those up to the age of 16, and 'adolescents' and 'young people' interchangeably to mean people between the ages of 16 and 18.

The Mental Health Act 1983 applies to England and Wales. Wales has its own Code of Practice for the MHA, due to come into practice in October 2016. It has a section on children and young people.

The Mental Capacity Act 2005 applies to England and Wales, and the Lord Chancellor has a duty to consult with the Welsh Assembly in compiling its Code of Practice. Therefore the MCA Code of Practice applies to both countries.

Scotland and Northern Ireland have their own legislation.

Notes on individual chapters

In Chapter 2 the Human Rights Act 1998 is described. This is a significant piece of legislation which is having an impact at many levels of society. Although the principles of the European Convention on Human Rights were ratified by the UK in the 1950s, since the Human Rights Act became enshrined in UK law it has become much easier for individuals to draw attention to their rights when they are infringed and to seek redress. It also highlights the rights of children as individuals. This chapter includes a number of important cases heard in the courts that have had a direct effect on psychiatric practice.

Chapter 3 deals with the Children Act 1989 and its amendments of 2004. The main points are parental responsibility, the private and public law elements and why a child or young person might need to be assessed using this legal framework

Consent is covered in Chapter 4, with an emphasis on why you need it and how you get it. The Montgomery case is briefly described and the impact this may have on gaining consent. The rest of the chapter inspects the key cases that have been heard before the courts involving consent and refusal, and also surveys professional guidelines. Finally, there are some notes on decision-making concerning admission and treatment.

Chapter 5 deals with confidentiality and its limits (which, it turns out, are many) in the doctor–patient relationship. Clinicians need to be aware of the professional guidelines and also the seemingly broadening definitions of the public interest.

In Chapter 6 the MHA is summarised. There is no lower age limit in using the MHA to detain a patient, and a case has recently been published illustrating its use with an 8-year-old child (Thomas *et al*, 2015). Figures showing how widely the MHA is used with children and young people are hard to find.

It should be mentioned here that, although not directly concerning the MHA, the confusing term 'zone of parental control' only ever appeared in the 2008 version of the MHA Code of Practice for England (but not in that for Wales). In the current version of the Code (Department of Health, 2015) it has been replaced by the more restrained term 'scope of parental responsibility', which I mention in Chapters 2 and 4. Viewed against the background of the increasing recognition of children's human rights, this concept appears to be highly questionable, particularly for children who lack competence and are, by definition, the most vulnerable. These are the children whose mental disorder does not warrant using the MHA and who fall into the gap left between the MHA and either the Children's Act or the MCA.

But all this looks set to change as a result of the Law Commission review (Law Commission, 2015) and the replacement of the deprivation of liberty safeguards with something else. We can only hope that it does not make things more complicated.

Other topics discussed in Chapter 6 are section 131 of the MHA and the highly publicised use of section 136 when it has led to detentions of children and young people in police cells. Of equivalent political importance is the great difficulty clinicians face in finding beds for children and young people needing urgent in-patient care (Faculty of Child and Adolescent Psychiatry, 2015a). The resulting placement of children with mental disorders in states of distress and risk at great distance from their homes has seemed to many clinicians to be an outrage.

In Chapter 7 the MCA is outlined. Its applicability to young people is limited to 16- and 17-year-olds and the now notorious deprivation of liberty safeguards (DoLS) cannot be used for anyone under 18. Clinicians need to know about the principles of this Act, capacity assessments and also the interaction between this Act and the MHA.

Finally, Chapter 8 considers aspects of juvenile justice. It includes information about secure accommodation and restraint, and an overview of the points of contact a young person known to CAMHS might have with the criminal justice system. The so-called forensic sections of the MHA are outlined at the end.

This book has been written to meet the needs of practising clinicians, who often have to make decisions in situations of complexity. However, it cannot tell clinicians what to do in particular circumstances and, of course, it will only be up to date until the next change in the law. References are given to enable readers to explore other sources of information, should they have the time to do so. My intention has been to make the subject, in the words of Dickens's Mr Kenge, plain and to the purpose:

> 'It could not, sir,' said Mr Kenge, 'have been stated more plainly and to the purpose, if it had been a case at law.'
> 'Did you ever know English law, or equity either, plain and to the purpose?' said my guardian.
>
> (Charles Dickens, *Bleak House*, 1852–1853).

CHAPTER 2

The rights of the child

The European Convention on Human Rights (ECHR) was drawn up in the wake of the Second World War and was signed by the UK government in 1950. However, the Convention did not form part of UK law until the Human Rights Act 1998 came into effect in October 2000.

The European Court of Human Rights was established in 1959 in Strasbourg to protect the Convention rights. Since the Human Rights Act came into effect in 2000, individuals have been able to take cases to the UK courts instead of Strasbourg. It is unlawful for a public body (and this includes Social Services, the National Health Service (NHS) and clinicians treating patients on behalf of the State) to act in a way that is incompatible with a Convention right (see Zigmond & Brindle, 2016: p. 9). It is the duty of all UK courts, including the Supreme Court, to interpret legislation so that it is compatible with the ECHR. If the court decides that it is not possible to interpret legislation so that it is compatible with the Convention it will issue a 'declaration of incompatibility'.

So what do clinicians in child and adolescent mental health services (CAMHS) need to know about this legislation? It is of course important to have an appreciation of the articles and some of the related cases heard in law that have shaped contemporary psychiatric practice. Article 5 in particular, as discussed in Chapter 1, is having a significant impact on the management of many patients who may now fall into the category of people, including children and adolescents, who would be considered to be deprived of their liberty. And finally the idea of competing rights, demonstrated in the case of Axon (see p. 20), also needs to be borne in mind. But above all, an important effect that this legislation is having is to emphasise that children have rights too.

Several breaches of human rights legislation by the UK are worthy of mention. The UK was found to be in breach of Articles 5 and 6 in the case of *T v United Kingdom (Application 24724/94)* [2000] (see below); and the so-called Bournewood case (*HL v UK* (2004)) was found to breach Article 5 rights. This led to the incorporation of the Deprivation of Liberty Safeguards into the Mental Capacity Act 2005. The MCA came into force in 2007 and the DoLS safeguards in 2009. This is discussed further in Chapters 1 and 7.

Interestingly for psychiatrists, the first case in which an Act of Parliament was deemed incompatible with human rights legislation involved detention under the Mental Health Act 1983 (MHA) in *R (on the application of H) v Mental Health Review Tribunal, North & East London Region & Anor* [2001]. The arguments are quite technical and concern the meaning of section 72 of the MHA in the application to a mental health tribunal. The patient in effect argued that the burden of proof (wrongly) fell upon him to demonstrate that the criteria for admission were not satisfied, whereas he felt he should be entitled to be discharged if it could not be demonstrated that the criteria for his continuing detention were met. As Article 5 (see below) requires the public authority to prove that the patient is of unsound mind, this appeal was allowed and a declaration of incompatibility with Article 5 was made. As a result, hospitals now must demonstrate the lawfulness of continuing detention before the tribunal hearing occurs.

The Human Rights Act imposes another layer of legal requirements on common law and statute law. The most relevant articles for children's mental health are outlined below. A good guide to the Act is available from the Department for Constitutional Affairs (2006). It includes a list of the Act's sections and articles, as well as examples from case law to demonstrate its application.

There are three types of Article:

▶ those with an absolute prohibition (Articles 3, 12 and 14)
▶ those with an absolute prohibition but subject to exceptions (Articles 2 and 5)
▶ those where the individual's right must be balanced against the rights of others or of society (Articles 8, 9 and 10).

In addition:

▶ the right must be specified, i.e. precisely delineated by the court
▶ the court needs to consider the extent to which the right imposes a positive obligation on the State
▶ where balancing is required, several factors must be considered, such as the rule of law, legitimate aims and proportionality
▶ there is a margin of appreciation in recognition that States may implement public policy according to local needs and conditions

(see Kennedy & Grubb, 2000: pp. 31–35).

The Human Rights Act concerns actions undertaken by public bodies. As explained by Zigmond & Brindle (2016: p. 9), clinicians must abide by the Act when treating an NHS patient or a private patient on behalf of the State. In the next section I discuss the articles likely to be of most relevance to CAMHS clinicians (note that the article numbers are the same for the ECHR and the Human Rights Act).

Convention articles

Article 2: Right to life

1. Everyone's right to life shall be protected by law. No one shall be deprived of his life intentionally save in the execution of a sentence of a court following his conviction of a crime for which this penalty is provided by law.
2. Deprivation of life shall not be regarded as inflicted in contravention of this article when it results from the use of force which is no more than absolutely necessary:
   a. in defence of any person from unlawful violence;
   b. in order to effect a lawful arrest or to prevent escape of a person lawfully detained;
   c. in action lawfully taken for the purpose of quelling a riot or insurrection.

Hospitals are under a duty to take positive steps to safeguard a patient's right to life (Department for Constitutional Affairs, 2006). This does not include a right to take your own life, and so hospitals must protect patients from suicide. Two cases are worthy of discussion here. Although they concern adult patients, they have clear implications for the clinical care of younger patients.

First is the Savage case (Jackson, 2013: p. 335; Zigmund & Brindle, 2016: p. 18). In *Savage v South Essex Partnership NHS Foundation Trust* [2008] the House of Lords decided that there had been a breach of Article 2 rights when a detained adult patient, Carol Savage, absconded from a ward and took her own life. The responsibility therefore lies with hospitals to ensure that proper systems are in place to protect patients from their own actions.

However, in the words of Lord Rodger:

'The operational obligation arises only if members of staff know or ought to know that a particular patient presents real and immediate risk of suicide. In these circumstances article 2 requires them to do all that can reasonably be expected to prevent the patient from committing suicide.'

The case makes salutary reading for all psychiatrists from the point of view of standards of care, risk assessments and the implementation of hospital policies on levels of observation. In a later claim for damages concerning this case (*Savage v South Essex Partnership NHS Foundation Trust* [2010] Mr Justice Mackay commented:

'It is easy to see these documents as tiresome management-driven bureaucracy, as I fear Dr A did, as to an extent did I on first introduction to them, but as the case progressed I saw more clearly what an important role they could play in circumstances such as these.'

Several years later, in 2012 the Supreme Court considered a similar case, but this time involving an informally admitted adult, Melanie Rabone (Jackson, 2013: p. 336). The judgment can be found in *Rabone & Anor v Pennine Care NHS Foundation* [2012]. The patient had been admitted following a number of suicide attempts and was thought to be at moderately high risk of further attempts. She was granted a weekend's home leave following a meeting with her and her mother, and she took her life during that leave. Her parents brought a civil negligence claim and a claim for damages against the hospital trust for breaching their daughter's Article 2 right to life. The trust admitted negligence, but the claim for damages was disallowed.

In Lord Dyson's judgment (paragraphs 28–34) there is a debate about the difference between informal and detained patients and the operational obligations of the hospital trust in this case:

'As regards the differences between an informal psychiatric patient and one who is detained under the MHA, these are in many ways more apparent than real.

[...]

The very reason why she was admitted was because there was a risk that she would commit suicide from which she needed to be protected.

[...]

I am in no doubt that the trust owed the operational duty to her to take reasonable steps to protect her from the real and immediate risk of suicide. [...] Although she was not a detained patient, it is clear that, if she had insisted on leaving the hospital, the authorities could and should have exercised their powers under the MHA to prevent her from doing so. [...] In reality, the difference between her position and that of a hypothetical detained psychiatric patient, who (apart from the fact of being detained) was in circumstances similar to those of Melanie, would have been one of form, not substance.'

And from Lady Hale:

'There is a difficult balance to be struck between the right of the individual patient to freedom and self-determination and her right to be prevented from taking her own life. She wanted to go home and her doctor thought that it would be good for her to begin to take responsibility for herself. He was obviously wrong about that, but was he so wrong that the hospital is to be held in breach of her human rights for failing to protect her? It may not always be enough simply to say that the experts were agreed that the decision to give her home leave was one which no reasonable psychiatrist would have taken. But in this case it also appears that there was no proper assessment of the risks before she was given leave and no proper planning for her care during the leave.'

So much for adult patients, but what about adolescents? Clearly these arguments are even more difficult for younger patients, and the court struggles in trying to balance the right of adolescents to autonomy against its desire to protect them from acts that may cause them harm. This tension is dealt with more fully in Chapter 3 in the difficult area of adolescents' refusal of treatment.

Article 2 then poses an obligation on all public authorities, including the courts, to preserve life. The court may conceivably find that, in order to exercise its inherent jurisdiction, its duty in this respect cannot be ignored when it comes to saving the life of a seriously ill adolescent (for further discussion see Fortin (2014) and Jackson (2013: p. 263)). Adolescents who refuse treatment have a number of competing Convention rights, among them a right to life under Article 2. This may emerge as a solution to the difficult problem of adolescent refusal of medical treatment in the future.

Article 3: Prohibition of torture

No one shall be subjected to torture or to inhuman or degrading treatment or punishment.

The principle case to be considered in relation to Article 3 is *Herczegfalvy v Austria* (1992), although this was heard in the European Court of Human Rights. This case concerned a mentally ill patient who was detained, handcuffed to his bed and allegedly administered antipsychotics and food, measures that were pronounced therapeutically necessary and considered to be within normal practice at that time in that country. The judgment stated:

> 'As a general rule, such a measure would not be inhuman or degrading so long as the Court was satisfied that the medical necessity had been convincingly shown to exist. In the instant case, despite the continued usage of restraints, the evidence before the Court was not sufficient to disprove the government's argument of necessity. It followed that no violation of Article 3 had occurred.'

So, medical necessity was demonstrated, and the European Court found that no violation of Article 3 had occurred.

The change of the law in the UK such that approved clinicians and responsible clinicians no longer need to be doctors to be in charge of a detained patient (see Chapter 6) raises some interesting questions about who calls what a 'medical necessity'. It seems likely that some challenges will arise in the future on this basis. The use of force and restraint also needs to be considered within this Article: neither must interfere with a patient's rights. Restraint policies are discussed in detail in the new MHA Code of Practice (Department of Health, 2015) and I also refer to them in Chapter 8.

Article 5: Right to liberty and security of person

1 Everyone has the right to liberty and security of person. No one shall be deprived of his liberty save in the following cases and in accordance with a procedure prescribed by law:

 a. the lawful detention of a person after conviction by a competent court;

 b. the lawful arrest or detention of a person for non-compliance with the lawful

---

order of a court or in order to secure the fulfilment of any obligation prescribed by law;

c. the lawful arrest or detention of a person effected for the purpose of bringing him before the competent legal authority on reasonable suspicion of having committed an offence or when it is reasonably considered necessary to prevent his committing an offence or fleeing after having done so;

d. the detention of a minor by lawful order for the purpose of educational supervision or his lawful detention for the purpose of bringing him before the competent legal authority;

e. the lawful detention of persons for the prevention of the spreading of infectious diseases, of persons of unsound mind, alcoholics or drug addicts, or vagrants;

f. the lawful arrest or detention of a person to prevent his effecting an unauthorised entry into the country or of a person against whom action is being taken with a view to deportation or extradition.

2. Everyone who is arrested shall be informed promptly, in a language which he understands, of the reasons for his arrest and of any charge against him.

3. Everyone arrested or detained in accordance with the provisions of paragraph 1c. of this Article shall be brought promptly before a judge or other officer authorised by law to exercise judicial power and shall be entitled to trial within a reasonable time or to release pending trial. Release may be conditioned by guarantees to appear for trial.

4. Everyone who is deprived of his liberty by arrest or detention shall be entitled to take proceedings by which the lawfulness of his detention shall be decided speedily by a court and his release ordered if the detention is not lawful.

5. Everyone who has been the victim of arrest or detention in contravention of the provisions of this Article shall have an enforceable right to compensation.

Article 5 has become important for psychiatrists for several reasons. The first is the need to demonstrate objective medical evidence when detaining a person of unsound mind. The second is the important role that the mental health tribunal fulfils in acting as the independent body, as it were, for assessing whether continued detention of a patient is necessary, as required under Article 5. The third is the question of what constitutes a deprivation of liberty. I will describe the first and the third of these in more detail here.

When detaining persons of unsound mind, the significant case from the European Court of Human Rights is *Winterwerp v The Netherlands* (1979). Concerning the need for objective medical evidence, the judgment stated (emphasis added):

> 'In the court's opinion [...] the individual concerned should not be deprived of his liberty unless he has been reliably shown to be of 'unsound mind'. The very nature of what has to be established before the competent national authority – that is, a true mental disorder – calls for *objective medical expertise*. Further, the mental disorder must be of a kind or degree warranting compulsory confinement. What is more, *the validity of continued confinement depends upon the persistence of such a disorder.*'

Two points need to be borne in mind here. First is the need to keep the person's mental state under review, as continued detention can only be justified if the need for it persists. Second, in light of the fact that approved clinicians and responsible clinicians no longer need to be doctors (see above and Chapter 6), whether the courts will accept such testimonial from persons who are not medically qualified has yet to be tested.

The lawful deprivation of liberty of people with mental disorders who lack capacity but who need to be detained in their best interests is negotiated by use of the Deprivation of Liberty Safeguards (DoLS). These were issued as an addition to the Mental Capacity Act as a result of a breach of human rights legislation (I discuss this in Chapters 1 and 7). However, DoLS only apply to people over 18 years of age. So where do we stand in the case of children and adolescents?

An important case much discussed has been *Neilsen v Denmark* (1988), which concerned a 12-year-old boy admitted to a children's psychiatric ward for several months. The issue under question was whether this amounted to a deprivation of liberty in the meaning of Article 5 of the ECHR: the conclusion was that it did not. Much, it seemed, depended on the 'concrete situation', a term drawn from another notable case, *Guzzardi v Italy 7367/76* (1980), and encompassing all the factors that needed to be taken into account in the context and setting of the case.

Another case to consider, this time in the UK, is that of *A Local Authority v A (a child) & Anor* [2010] in the family division of the High Court. The question before the court was whether the circumstances of the child's domestic care constituted a deprivation of liberty, thus engaging Article 5, and what role the local authority had played in this.

The case concerned A, an 8-year-old child with significant learning disability, looked after at home by her family. As part of her ordinary care she was locked in her room at night. Drawing on several previous cases concerning the deprivation of liberty, Mr Justice Munby (as he was then) described how the three following conditions were used to test whether this was a deprivation of liberty:

'i)   an objective element of 'a person's confinement to a certain limited place for a not negligible length of time';
ii)   a subjective element, namely that the person has not 'validly consented to the confinement in question'; and
iii) the deprivation of liberty must be one for which the State is responsible.'

The judgment concluded that A was not deprived of her liberty within the meaning of the Article. As for the role of the local authority, Mr Justice Munby said:

'Where the State – here, a local authority – knows or ought to know that a vulnerable child or adult is subject to restrictions on their liberty by a private individual that arguably give rise to a deprivation of liberty, then its positive obligations under Article 5 will be triggered.
[...] These will include the duty to investigate.'

He goes on to stipulate that subsequent actions will depend on the context, and that reasonable and proportionate measures should be taken.

We might reasonably have concluded from this that the court has been somewhat reluctant to see restrictions of liberty as deprivation of liberty, especially when someone with parental responsibility is in support of the arrangements. As Lord Justice Thorpe said in *RK (by her litigation friend, the Official Solicitor) v BCC & Ors* [2011]:

> 'The consensus is to this effect: The decisions of the European Court of Human Rights in *Neilsen v Denmark* (1988) 11 EHRR 175 and of this court in *Re K* [2002] 2 WLR 1141 demonstrate that an adult in the exercise of parental responsibility may impose, or may authorise others to impose, restrictions on the liberty of the child. However restrictions so imposed must not in their totality amount to deprivation of liberty. Deprivation of liberty engages the art 5 rights of the child and a parent may not lawfully detain or authorise the deprivation of liberty of a child.'

But this was before Cheshire West.

In a case heard recently (*Re D (A Child: Deprivation of liberty)* (2015)) a hospital submitted an application seeking a declaration that the deprivation of a child's liberty was lawful. This followed the outcome of the decision of the Supreme Court in *Surrey County Council v P, Cheshire West and Chester Council v P* [2014] (known as the Cheshire West case, which I discuss further in Chapter 1). The child, known as D, was a 15-year-old with diagnoses of attention-deficit hyperactivity disorder, Tourette syndrome and Asperger syndrome who demonstrated challenging behaviours at home. He had been admitted informally to hospital in October 2013. At the time of the court case, in March 2015, he was still an in-patient, despite now being considered fit for discharge. The practical difficulty had been in finding a suitable residential placement for him.

The questions before the court, presided over by Mr Justice Keehan, was whether this constituted a deprivation of liberty that would engage Article 5; whether the parents could consent to what would otherwise be a deprivation of liberty; and if not, whether the court should exercise its powers under its inherent jurisdiction to declare this deprivation of liberty lawful and in D's best interests. Mr Justice Keehan is mindful of Cheshire West and that, after the age of 16, the situation for D would need to be clarified in the Court of Protection. However, he tried to find a path between the rocks. In his judgment, he considered that D lived in conditions at the hospital that did indeed amount to a deprivation of liberty. But he then said:

> 'The decision to keep an autistic 15 year old boy who has erratic, challenging and potentially harmful behaviours under constant supervision and control is a quite different matter; to do otherwise would be neglectful. In such a case I consider the decision to keep this young person under constant supervision and control is the proper exercise of parental responsibility.
>
> [...]
>
> I am satisfied that, on the particular facts of this case, the consent of D's parents to his placement at Hospital B, with all of the restrictions placed upon his life there, falls within the 'zone of parental responsibility'. In the exercise of their parental responsibility for D, I am satisfied they have and are able to consent to his placement.'

(For comments on the 'zone of parental responsibility' see Chapters 1 and 4.) In this case, the finding that parental sanction can authorise a deprivation of liberty, which appeared to hinge on the boy's disabilities, might well be seen by some to be inconsistent with the spirit of Cheshire West.

So what is a deprivation of liberty now?

The new Code of Practice for the MHA (Department of Health, 2015) in its general guidance says:

> '13.44 The precise scope of the term 'deprivation of liberty' is not fixed. In its 19 March judgment P v Cheshire West and Chester Council and another and P and Q v Surrey County Council ('Cheshire West'), the Supreme Court clarified that there is a deprivation of liberty in circumstances where a person is under continuous control and supervision, is not free to leave and lacks capacity to consent to these arrangements.
>
> 13.45 The Supreme Court also noted that factors which are not relevant in determining whether there is a deprivation of liberty include the person's compliance or lack of objection and the reason or purpose behind a particular placement. The relative normality of the placement (whatever the comparison made) is also not relevant.
>
> 13.46 A deprivation of liberty can occur in domestic settings where the State is responsible for such arrangements. In such cases, an order should be sought from the Court of Protection.
>
> 13.47 The definition of a deprivation of liberty develops over time in accordance with the case law of the European Court of Human Rights and UK courts on article 5 of the ECHR. In order for decision-makers to be able to assess whether the situation they are faced with constitutes (or is likely to constitute) a deprivation of liberty, they should keep abreast of the latest case law developments.'

And in the chapter specifically on children and adolescents it gives the following advice:

> '19.48 Prior to the Supreme Court's judgment in Cheshire West, case law had established that persons with parental responsibility cannot authorise a deprivation of liberty. Cheshire West clarified the elements establishing a deprivation of liberty, but did not expressly decide whether a person with parental responsibility could, and if so in what circumstances, consent to restrictions that would, without their consent, amount to a deprivation of liberty. In determining whether a person with parental responsibility can consent to the arrangements which would, without their consent, amount to a deprivation of liberty, practitioners will need to consider and apply developments in case law following Cheshire West. In determining the limits of parental responsibility, decision-makers must carefully consider and balance: (i) the child's right to liberty under article 5, which should be informed by article 37 of the UNCRC, (ii) the parent's right to respect for the right to family life under article 8, which includes the concept of parental responsibility for the care and custody of minor children,

and (iii) the child's right to autonomy which is also protected under article 8. Decision makers should seek their own legal advice in respect of cases before them.'

It may be that further case law will help to clarify the position, but in the meantime new systems may be needed in our profession to help clinicians with these difficult cases. After all, such decisions are not normally part of the clinical task. The Law Society (2015*b*: pp. 94–105) has drawn up guidelines on identifying a deprivation of liberty in the under-18 age group but, as the Society is keen to point out, they do not constitute legal advice.

Article 6: Right to a fair trial

1. In the determination of his civil rights and obligations or of any criminal charge against him, everyone is entitled to a fair and public hearing within a reasonable time by an independent and impartial tribunal established by law. Judgment shall be pronounced publicly but the press and public may be excluded from all or part of the trial in the interest of morals, public order or national security in a democratic society, where the interests of juveniles or the protection of the private life of the parties so require, or to the extent strictly necessary in the opinion of the court in special circumstances where publicity would prejudice the interests of justice.
2. Everyone charged with a criminal offence shall be presumed innocent until proved guilty according to law.
3. Everyone charged with a criminal offence has the following minimum rights:
   a. to be informed promptly, in a language which he understands and in detail, of the nature and cause of the accusation against him;
   b. to have adequate time and facilities for the preparation of his defence;
   c. to defend himself in person or through legal assistance of his own choosing or, if he has not sufficient means to pay for legal assistance, to be given it free when the interests of justice so require;
   d. to examine or have examined witnesses against him and to obtain the attendance and examination of witnesses on his behalf under the same conditions as witnesses against him;
   e. to have the free assistance of an interpreter if he cannot understand or speak the language used in court.

In considering Article 6, two cases are worth mentioning.

In the case of *T v United Kingdom (Application 24724/94)* [2000], known more commonly as the case of Thompson and Venables, who killed the 2-year-old James Bulger, it was found by the European Court of Human Rights that Article 6 had been breached. It was considered that one of the two 10-year-old boys involved had not received a fair hearing. It was found that he was unable to participate effectively in the 3-week trial in public in a Crown Court, and that in future such trials involving serious offences with high levels of media and public interest should be held in such a way that the child's feelings of inhibition and intimidation should be reduced.

The court also found that the way the sentence was fixed by the Secretary of State rather than by an impartial tribunal breached this Article.

Competing rights also need to be considered. This was demonstrated in *R (on the application of B) v Stafford Combined Court* [2006] and is described by Jackson (2013: p. 369). In this case, the right to a fair trial of an adult defendant (Article 6) conflicted with the right to confidentiality of a 14-year-old girl (Article 8). The girl was the main prosecution witness in the trial of the man, who was subsequently convicted of sexually abusing her. His legal representatives had requested access to her medical records (she had a history of attempting suicide), arguing that they were relevant to her credibility as a witness. The girl was not represented in court and the conduct of the judge was criticised. The court itself was found to have breached the girl's Article 8 rights (see below).

Finally, and of relevance to both Articles 5 and 6, it should be noted that if patients detained under the MHA are dependent on a mental health tribunal to argue against detention then, as Zigmond & Brindle (2016: pp. 14–15) point out, it cannot be fair that the burden of bringing the appeal falls on an unwell person, be it an adult or an adolescent. It seems likely that this will be found to be incompatible with Article 5 rights.

Article 8: Right to respect for private and family life

1. Everyone has the right to respect for his private and family life, his home and his correspondence.
2. There shall be no interference by a public authority with the exercise of this right except such as is in accordance with the law and is necessary in a democratic society in the interests of national security, public safety or the economic well-being of the country, for the prevention of disorder or crime, for the protection of health or morals, or for the protection of the rights and freedoms of others.

Article 8 encompasses various rights relevant to psychiatric practice, such as non-consensual treatment, smoking bans, seclusion, restraint, access to medical records and family visiting. It might even, as suggested by Barber *et al* (2012: p. 131) include being kept on a treatment waiting list. But it is a qualified right. In practice, if a (medical) intervention can be shown to be necessary and intended for the protection of health, then the protection offered against breaching this Article is qualified (Jackson, 2013: p. 337). This has been borne out in case law. For example, in *R (on the application of N) v M & Ors* [2002] it was stipulated that if the treatment can be convincingly shown to be medically necessary then neither Article 3 nor Article 8 will be violated, since the interference will be proportionate and justified.

Might Article 8 affect parents? In the interesting case of *R (on the application of Axon) v Secretary of State for Health* [2006], a mother applied for judicial review of Department of Health guidance on reproductive health for under-16-year-olds. She argued that the guidance, which clarified that individuals under the age of 16 could expect confidential advice about contraception and abortion, was not lawful (see Chapter 4) and that, in excluding parents from important decisions concerning their children, it infringed her right to respect for her family life under Article 8.

This has been seen as a post-Human Rights Act challenge to the Gillick case. The court, presided over by Mr Justice Silber, denied the claim. In so doing, he quoted Lord Scarman's judgment in *Gillick* (this is also quoted in Chapter 4 of this book) and went on to suggest:

> 'a parental right yields to the young person's right to make his own decisions when the young person reaches a sufficient understanding and intelligence to be capable of making up his or her mind in relation to the matter requiring decision, and this autonomy of a young person must undermine any Article 8 rights of a parent to family life.'

And what about children themselves? In *Re Roddy (a child) (identification: restriction on publication) Torbay Borough Council v News Group Newspapers* [2004], in the context of confidentiality, Mr Justice Munby (as he then was) confirmed that Article 8 applies to minors in a qualified sense. Its application is dependent on the child's maturity in the sense articulated in *Gillick*, but in addition he said:

> 'A child is, of course, as much entitled to the protection of the Convention – and specifically of Articles 8 and 10 – as anyone else. But [...] the personal autonomy guaranteed by Article 8 (and, I would add, by Article 10) is necessarily somewhat qualified in the case of a child. For, depending on the circumstances, decision-making power may rest not with the child but with the child's parents or even with the court.'

From Europe to the United Nations

The UN Convention on the Rights of the Child

Unlike the ECHR (via the Human Rights Act), the UN Convention on the Rights of the Child 1989, known also as the UNCRC or the CRC, is not legally enforced in the UK, but was ratified by the UK in 1991. However, the Convention has an important role internationally in uniting governments to recognise the status of children.

According to the UNICEF website:

> 'These rights describe what a child needs to survive, grow, and live up to their potential in the world. The Convention has 54 articles that cover all aspects of a child's life and set out the civil, political, economic, social and cultural rights that all children everywhere are entitled to' (UNICEF, 2016).

The UNCRC has been signed by 194 of the world's 196 countries. At the time of writing, only Somalia (with no acting government) and the USA are not signatories. The fact that the USA has not signed has attracted some debate. Fortin (2014), for example, suggests that this might be because the USA takes its obligations seriously and recognises the major flaws in the

Convention: namely, that it is aspirational and that there is no mechanism of enforcement. Some of the countries that have ratified it have expressed reservations, as would be expected. The UK has also attracted criticism from writers such as Fortin for its repeated failure to implement the aims of the Convention, particularly in the areas of juvenile justice, and specifically the age of criminal responsibility (discussed further in Chapter 8).

Four articles of the UNCRC are seen as especially relevant in helping the interpretation of other articles. These concern non-discrimination (Article 2); the best interests of the child (Article 3): the right to life, survival and development (Article 6): and the right to be heard (Article 12).

Many of the other articles are also relevant to children's mental health and the reader is referred to the UNICEF website (www.unicef.org.uk/UNICEFs-Work/UN-Convention) for a complete schedule. The articles most relevant to juvenile justice are 3, 37 and 40, and these are reproduced in Chapter 8.

The UN Convention on the Rights of Persons with Disabilities

This Convention, which came into operation in 2008, also attracted a large number of signatories (160 by July 2016). It follows work by the UN on changing attitudes and approaches to people with disabilities and comprises 50 articles. Article 7 concerns children with disabilities. Article 13, concerning access to justice, and Article 14, on liberty and security of person, are also relevant to children's mental health.

Conclusion

The European Convention on Human Rights, the Human Rights Act and the UN Convention on the Rights of Persons with Disabilities can all be seen to emphasise the rights of children and young people as individuals. Some of the cases arising in the courts as a consequence of this legislation have had a direct effect on the practice of psychiatry (and therefore child psychiatry). The particular issue of ECHR Article 5 rights, and the working definition of what constitutes a deprivation of liberty, have greatly exercised clinicians and the courts, and further developments in the field are awaited.

CHAPTER 3

The Children Act 1989 and the 2004 amendments

The Children Act 1989 was intended to bring together various pieces of legislation about children and to assimilate private law with public law.

Phrases from the original 1989 Act such as a child in need, significant harm and the welfare checklist have become part of the lexicon of child and adolescent psychiatry. Safeguarding was a word not commonly in use until enshrined in amendments introduced by the Children Act 2004. Although the Children Act 2004 exists, it was an Act of amendment and the current legislation is the Children Act 1989 (as amended in 2004).

Clinicians will come into contact with the Act in several ways. Primarily they will need to know who has parental responsibility for a child or young person. Without knowing this, the basis of consent for any interventions is unclear. Knowledge of the Act is also necessary when encountering any forms of abuse in children. It becomes essential in dealing with difficult emergencies, for example knowing the social care responsibilities of local authorities and when a section 25 secure order might be indicated. In any services where children and young people with mental health problems also have particularly complex family situations (on in-patient units, for example), knowledge of the Act is important, and clinicians acting as professional or expert witnesses will also need a reasonable working knowledge of it.

It should be noted that, although children and young people up to the age of 18 can be detained using section 25 of the Children Act (see below), this does not authorise treatment. If the main purpose of the intervention is assessment and treatment, then it is more appropriate to use the Mental Health Act 1983 (see Chapter 6). If the child is behaviourally disturbed and the purpose is containment of the behaviour rather than assessment and treatment, then a secure order using section 25 of the Children Act may be more appropriate. Secure orders are discussed further in Chapter 8.

This chapter will not cover care and adoption proceedings, as these are beyond the scope of this book and are not specific to the field of children's mental health.

It is relevant to mention a few other pieces of legislation since the enactment of the Children Act 1989 and its amendments from 2004.

These include the Children and Young Persons Act 2008, which relates principally to children in the care system, and the Children and Families Act 2014. The Children and Young Persons Act applies to England and Wales and was intended to improve the stability of placements and educational attainment. It need not concern us further here. The Children and Families Act 2014 includes provisions for adoption and contact, and introduces child arrangements orders in place of what used to be known as the section 8 orders – resident and contact orders. It also introduces new controls over the expert witness, and describes the new education, health and care plans (EHCPs), which many clinicians will by now have heard about. The Children and Families Act has also introduced a clause into the Children Act 1989 that encourages the court to presume, unless the contrary is shown, that involvement of each parent in the life of the child will benefit the child's welfare. There are new provisions too for the assessment of young carers and parent carers.

Although the Children Act covers both England and Wales, there are some differences in the detailed provisions in the two countries. When published, the aim of the 1989 Act was:

An Act to reform the law relating to children; to provide for local authority services for children in need and others; to amend the law with respect to children's homes, community homes, voluntary homes and voluntary organisations; to make provision with respect to fostering, child minding and day care for young children and adoption; and for connected purposes.
[16th November 1989]

(The Children Act 1989: Chapter 41)

The 2004 Act of amendment has as its purpose:

An Act to make provision for the establishment of a Children's Commissioner; to make provision about services provided to and for children and young people by local authorities and other persons; to make provision in relation to Wales about advisory and support services relating to family proceedings; to make provision about private fostering, child minding and day care, adoption review panels, the defence of reasonable punishment, the making of grants as respects children and families, child safety orders, the Children's Commissioner for Wales, the publication of material relating to children involved in certain legal proceedings and the disclosure by the Inland Revenue of information relating to children.
[15th November 2004]

(The Children Act 2004: Chapter 31)

An overview of the Children Act 1989

The Act applies to all children and young people up to the age of 18. It gives a prominent role to parents and especially to the mother, abolishing the rule of law that a father is the natural guardian of his child, which may be unpalatable for individuals of some traditionally male-oriented cultural groups. It uses the language of responsibilities rather than rights.

The main principles are:

- ▶ the child's welfare is paramount
- ▶ the court shall have regard to the welfare checklist (see below)
- ▶ delay in resolving questions about upbringing should be avoided
- ▶ an order (for example, with whom the child should live) should be made only if that is better than no order at all.

The main parts of the Act relating to children's mental health law are shown in Table 3.1 and outlined in more detail in the sections that follow.

Table 3.1 The main parts of the Children Act 1989 (as amended in 2004) relating to children's mental health law

Part and section	Notes
Part I Introductory	
Section 1	Welfare of the child
Sections 2–4	Parental responsibility
Part II Orders with respect to children in family proceedings	
Section 8	Residence, contact and other orders (known as part 8 orders, but see notes in the text)
Part III Local authority support for children and families	
Section 17	Provision of services for children in need
Section 20	Provision of accommodation for children
Section 25	Use of accommodation for restricting liberty
Section 27	Cooperation between authorities
Part IV Care and supervision	
Section 31	Care and supervision orders
Section 36	Education supervision orders
Part V Protection of children	
Section 43	Child assessment orders
Section 44	Orders for emergency protection of children
Section 47	Local authority's duty to investigate

Part I: introductory

The welfare checklist

A court shall have regard in particular to:

(a) the ascertainable wishes and feelings of the child concerned (considered in the light of his age and understanding);

(b) his physical, emotional and educational needs;

(c) the likely effect on him of any change in his circumstances;

(d) his age, sex, background and any characteristics of his which the court considers relevant;

(e) any harm which he has suffered or is at risk of suffering;

(f) how capable each of his parents, and any other person in relation to whom the court considers the question to be relevant, is of meeting his needs;

(g) the range of powers available to the court under this Act in the proceedings in question.

(Children Act 1989: Part 1, section 1(3))

Sections 2, 3 and 4 of Part I outline what is meant by parental responsibility.

Parental responsibility

To simplify matters, I show here only selected sections from Part I. I have omitted, for example, details concerning cases where children have been conceived by artificial means. It may be worth noting that parents who do not have parental responsibility may yet have a role in participating in treatment decisions according to European Court of Human Rights legislation.

From Part I:

'(1) In this Act "parental responsibility" means all the rights, duties, powers, responsibilities and authority which by law a parent of a child has in relation to the child and his property.'

'(5) A person who –

(a) does not have parental responsibility for a particular child; but

(b) has care of the child,

may (subject to the provisions of this Act) do what is reasonable in all the circumstances of the case for the purpose of safeguarding or promoting the child's welfare.'

And main points about this are:

'(1) Where a child's father and mother were married to each other at the time of his birth, they shall each have parental responsibility for the child.

(2) Where a child's father and mother were not married to each other at the time of his birth –

   (a) the mother shall have parental responsibility for the child;

   (b) the father shall have parental responsibility for the child if he has acquired it (and has not ceased to have it) in accordance with the provisions of this Act [see below].

(3) References in this Act to a child whose father and mother were, or (as the case may be) were not, married to each other at the time of his birth must be read with section 1 of the Family Law Reform Act 1987 (which extends their meaning).

(4) The rule of law that a father is the natural guardian of his legitimate child is abolished.

(5) More than one person may have parental responsibility for the same child at the same time.

(6) A person who has parental responsibility for a child at any time shall not cease to have that responsibility solely because some other person subsequently acquires parental responsibility for the child.

(7) Where more than one person has parental responsibility for a child, each of them may act alone and without the other (or others) in meeting that responsibility.'

So, the father who was not married to the mother at the time of the child's birth can acquire parental responsibility by:

▶ becoming registered on the birth certificate (after 1 December 2003 or the dates below if the child is born elsewhere in the UK)

▶ making a parental responsibility agreement with the mother which is registered with the court

▶ by means of a court order

(see Harbour, 2008: p. 36; British Medical Association (BMA), 2010).

For births in different parts of the UK the BMA (2010) has a useful summary:

▶ If the birth is registered in England, Wales or Northern Ireland, the father has parental responsibility if he is married to the mother at the time of the birth or subsequently. An unmarried father has parental responsibility if he is recorded on the child's birth certificate (at registration or on re-registration) from 1 December 2003 in England or Wales and from 15 April 2002 in Northern Ireland.

▶ If the birth is registered in Scotland, the father has parental responsibility if he is married to the mother at the time of the child's conception or subsequently. An unmarried father has parental responsibility if he is recorded on the child's birth certificate (at registration or on reregistration) from 4 May 2006.

▶ If the birth is registered outside the UK, the rules for the UK country where the child lives apply.

Can other people have parental responsibility?

Married step-parents and registered civil partners can acquire parental responsibility in the same ways as fathers (see above). Foster parents rarely have parental responsibility. Other people who can acquire parental responsibility for a child include:

▶ a guardian named in a will if no one with parental responsibility survives

▶ a guardian appointed by a court

▶ the adoptive parents, if a child is adopted

▶ a local authority (shared with anyone else with parental responsibility) while a child is subject to a care or supervision order

▶ for a child born under a surrogacy arrangement, the surrogate mother (and her husband, if she married) until the intended parents either obtain a parental order from a court under the Human Fertilisation and Embryology Act 1990 or adopt the child

(British Medical Association, 2010).

It is also possible for the court to have parental responsibility under either wardship or its inherent jurisdiction or by means of a section 8 order (see Chapter 4 for more on this).

Parents can, in addition, authorise another person, for example a teacher or childminder, to enact certain responsibilities or 'do what is reasonable', such as collecting medication or taking a child for an immunisation (Part I, section 3(5)).

In cases of disagreement between people with parental responsibility the BMA guidance suggests that an attempt at consensus should be made, but that the clinician can decide whether to proceed in spite of the disagreement. If, however, the procedure in question is irreversible, elective and controversial, doctors should seek legal advice and the authority of the court.

Case law has established that certain acts do need consensus between those with parental responsibility. These are:

▶ change of surname

▶ removal of the child from the jurisdiction

▶ serious or controversial medical treatment, except in an emergency

▶ decisions about education

▶ ritual (i.e. non-medical) circumcision

▶ immunisations

(see Kennedy & Grubb, 2000: p. 775; Puri et al, 2012: p. 197; Jackson, 2013: p. 257).

In Scotland the situation differs slightly: for any decision concerning a child anyone with parental responsibility must have regard to anyone else with those same responsibilities.

There is no requirement for doctors to communicate about ordinary medical treatment with an absent parent who has parental responsibility where the parents are not communicating with each other (British Medical Association, 2010).

Duration of parental responsibility

There is a slight difference of emphasis in this across the UK. In England, Wales and Northern Ireland, parental responsibilities may be exercised until a young person reaches 18 years of age. In Scotland, only those aspects of parental responsibility concerned with the giving of 'guidance' last until the age of 18. By guidance is meant advice. Other aspects of parental responsibility are lost at the age of 16, or earlier if the young person has acquired capacity to act on their own behalf (British Medical Association, 2010).

Part II, section 8: residence, contact and other orders

Section 8 orders, also known as private law orders, include prohibited steps orders, specific issue orders and what were called until quite recently contact orders and residence orders. The Children and Families Act 2014 has substituted contact and residence orders with child arrangements orders, which came into operation in April 2014.

Section 8 orders cannot be made (with the exception of what used to be called a residence order) for children who are on care orders (in the care of a local authority). In addition, again with the exception of a residence order, they do not last beyond the 16th birthday unless there are exceptional circumstances.

Prohibited steps orders

In cases where either contact with a particular person is considered harmful, or a child is at risk of being removed from the jurisdiction by one parent, the court can impose a prohibited steps order to prevent such situations occurring without its consent.

Specific issue orders

These are orders giving directions for the purpose of determining a specific question that has arisen, or that might arise, in connection with any aspect of parental responsibility for a child or young person. Specific medical treatments can be authorised by the court, for example.

Contact orders and residence orders

Before April 2014, the courts awarded contact orders and residence orders in cases where there were disputes between parents over a child's contact with the other parent or with whom the child was to live. These have now been replaced with child arrangements orders. It seems likely that the courts will specify on the new child arrangements orders the person with whom the child is to live and whether there will be any changes to parental responsibility for the duration of the order.

Examples of specific issues orders being used are given by Hale & Fortin (2010). These include giving blood to children and young people whose parents are Jehovah's Witnesses and the treatment of anorexia nervosa. However, in the case of the latter many psychiatrists would consider use of the Mental Health Act to be more appropriate.

Part III: the child in need

Section 17

According to section 17, a child is in need if:

'(a) the child is unlikely to achieve or maintain, or to have the opportunity of achieving or maintaining, a reasonable standard of health or development without the provision of services by a local authority under Part III of the Children Act 1989;

(b) the child's health or development is likely to be significantly impaired, or further impaired, without the provision of such services; or

(c) the child is disabled.'

And it is the duty of every local authority:

'(a) to safeguard and promote the welfare of children within their area who are in need; and

(b) so far as is consistent with that duty, to promote the upbringing of such children by their families by providing a range and level of services appropriate to those children's needs.'

It will be apparent to readers that many children and young people in CAMHS are children in need under these criteria. Under section 17, local authorities have responsibility for determining what services should be provided to such children, but this does not necessarily require local authorities themselves to be the service provider.

Section 20

Section 20 concerns the provision of accommodation for children in need under the age of 16, and stipulates that:

'(1) Every local authority shall provide accommodation for any child in need within their area who appears to them to require accommodation as a result of–

(a) there being no person who has parental responsibility for him;

(b) his being lost or having been abandoned; or

(c) the person who has been caring for him being prevented (whether or not permanently, and for whatever reason) from providing him with suitable accommodation or care.'

The caveats are that the wishes of the young person do need to be taken into account and that no one with parental responsibility objects.

Under section 21, the local authority also has a duty to accommodate children and young people who are removed or kept away from home, including those in police protection, in detention or on remand.

Section 25 deals with secure accommodation. Secure accommodation orders and the criteria for applying for them are discussed in more detail in Chapter 8. Although section 25 can provide authority to deprive a child of their liberty, it does not give any authority to provide medical treatment.

Section 27 imposes a duty on local authorities, local authority housing services and health bodies to cooperate with one another.

Part IV, section 31: care and supervision

Section 31 provides for care and supervision orders, known as public law orders. In the words of the Act:

'(1) On the application of any local authority or authorised person, the court may make an order –

(a) placing the child with respect to whom the application is made in the care of a designated local authority; or

(b) putting him under the supervision of a designated local authority

(2) A court may only make a care order or supervision order if it is satisfied –

(a) that the child concerned is suffering, or is likely to suffer, significant harm; and

(b) that the harm, or likelihood of harm, is attributable to –

(i) the care given to the child, or likely to be given to him if the order were not made, not being what it would be reasonable to expect a parent to give to him; or

(ii) the child's being beyond parental control.

(3) No care order or supervision order may be made with respect to a child who has reached the age of seventeen (or sixteen, in the case of a child who is married).'

Subsection (9) defines certain terms:

'"harm" means ill-treatment or the impairment of health or development including, in an amendment inserted after the publication of the Act for example, impairment suffered from seeing or hearing the ill-treatment of another;

"development" means physical, intellectual, emotional, social or behavioural development;

"health" means physical or mental health; and

"ill-treatment" includes sexual abuse and forms of ill-treatment which are not physical.'

And in subsection (10) it is explained that whether or not the harm is significant depends on comparing the child's health or development with that which could reasonably be expected of a similar child.

Care orders

A section 31 care order, which commits a child to the care of the local authority, can only be made up to the 17th birthday, but lasts until the child is 18. A care order cannot be made if the young person is over 16 and married. It can be ended by the young person, the local authority or someone with parental responsibility.

Supervision orders

A section 31 supervision order places a child or young person under the supervision of a social worker or probation officer, but does not confer parental responsibility. Under the terms of the order (and see Schedule 3 at the end of the Act, subsections 4 and 5 of which provide the detail), the child can be required to live in a particular place or participate in specified activities. Moreover, the supervised child can be required to attend for medical or psychiatric examination and treatment, although if they have sufficient understanding their consent is required.

Interim care or supervision orders

A section 38 interim order can be made if proceedings for a care order or a supervision order are adjourned. The court can give directions for a medical or psychiatric examination or other assessment of the child. However, if the child is of sufficient understanding to make an informed decision they may refuse to submit to examination or assessment. As a result of the Children and Families Act 2014, these orders can now be issued for longer than 28 days.

Education supervision orders

A local authority can apply for a section 36 education supervision order if they believe a child is not being properly educated.

Part V: child protection

Section 43

A section 43 child assessment order can be made if the court suspects that the child is suffering or likely to suffer harm, that this can only be determined by an assessment and that the assessment cannot be undertaken without an order.

Section 44

Section 44 concerns emergency protection orders. The court may make an emergency protection order if:

'(a) there is reasonable cause to believe that the child is likely to suffer significant harm if–

> (i) he is not removed to accommodation provided by or on behalf of the applicant; or
>
> (ii) he does not remain in the place in which he is then being accommodated.'

An emergency protection order may also be made if enquiries (for example, made under section 47) are being frustrated. This might occur if access to the child is unreasonably refused and the applicant believes that access is needed as a matter of urgency. The order gives authority to remove a child for protection for up to 8 days in the first instance. It also conveys parental responsibility. Additional powers can be granted, such as directions about contact with others and medical examinations. However, if a child or young person has sufficient understanding their consent is required for such directions.

Clinicians need to be aware of two cases in the past few years that have influenced the threshold for obtaining an emergency protection order. The first of these is *X Council v B (Emergency Protection Orders)* [2004]. From his review of the jurisprudence, Mr Justice Munby (as he then was) made 14 recommendations about the use of emergency protection orders, which he considered to be a 'draconian' and 'extremely harsh' measure, requiring 'exceptional justification' and 'extraordinarily compelling reasons'. He described how the 'imminent danger' that the child is supposed to be facing must be 'actually established' and how there should be 'scrupulous regard for the European Convention rights of both the child and the parents'. Furthermore, 'The evidence in support of the application for an EPO [emergency protection order] must be full, detailed, precise and compelling'.

In a subsequent case, *Re X (Emergency Protection Orders)* [2006], Mr Justice McFarlane (as he then was) considered that the principles elaborated by Mr Justice Munby should be applied at each application, and he made further recommendations. These included that the most recent case conference minutes should be available to the court, and that the following cases rarely, if ever, warrant an emergency protection order: emotional abuse; sexual abuse where the allegations are non-specific and where there is no evidence of immediate risk of harm to the child; and fabricated or induced illness, where there is no medical evidence of immediate risk of direct physical harm to the child.

Clinicians are therefore increasingly likely to hear of the alternatives to emergency protection orders, which are interim care orders under section 31 or child assessment orders under section 43.

Section 46

This allows for the removal of a child into police protection if it is believed that the child is at risk of significant harm. A child may not be kept in police protection for more than 72 hours.

Sections 38A and 44A

These sections refer to the so-called exclusion requirement, a provision that can be made in addition to an interim care order or emergency protection order to remove the perpetrator from the home, instead of having to remove the child.

Section 47

Section 47 describes the duty of the local authority to investigate immediately when a child in its area (a) is made the subject of an emergency protection order or is taken into police protection, (b) has contravened a ban imposed by a curfew notice under section 14 of the Crime and Disorder Act 1998, or (c) is at risk of significant harm. The local authority should instigate a core assessment to identify the needs of the child, and must ascertain the child's feelings and wishes as part of the assessment. A multi-agency strategy discussion should be convened to discuss any emergency action to be taken. This might include initiating proceedings for a section 31 supervision order, providing certain services or protecting the young person in some other way. For a more detailed discussion see *Working Together to Safeguard Children* (HM Government, 2015a).

What amendments did the 2004 Act bring in?

The Children Act 2004 swiftly followed the government report *Every Child Matters* (HM Treasury, 2003), and this in turn resulted from the inquiry conducted by Lord Laming into the death of Victoria Climbié. The focus of the amendments introduced by the 2004 Act was interagency working and accountability. It established the role of a Children's Commissioner for England, who has regard to the UNCRC (see Chapter 2). Section 11 emphasises the duties on a range of organisations and individuals in ensuring the need to safeguard and promote the welfare of children and prescribes how this should be done.

Although the welfare checklist in the original 1989 Act had suggested to professionals that, as far as possible, a young person's wishes and feelings are taken into account when considering use of the Act, this is emphasised more in the 2004 amendments. Thus, section 53 of the 2004 Act amends both sections 17 and 47 of the original 1989 Act, ensuring that before either section is used, the young person's wishes are listened to.

The scope is somewhat greater too: the amended Act now applies not only to children and young people under 18, but also to those aged 18–20 who have been looked after by a local authority after the age of 16, and to children or young people with an intellectual ('learning') disability.

Some of the other sections clinicians come across are as follows. Section 13 concerns the establishment of local safeguarding children boards (LSCBs) and section 14 describes their objectives. These replace area

Box 3.1 Statutory assessments under the Children Act 1989

- A child in need is defined under the Children Act 1989 as a child who is unlikely to achieve or maintain a reasonable level of health or development, or whose health and development is likely to be significantly or further impaired, without the provision of services; or a child who is disabled. Children in need may be assessed under section 17 of the Children Act 1989, in relation to their special educational needs, disabilities, as a carer, or because they have committed a crime. Where an assessment takes place, it will be carried out by a social worker. The process for assessment should also be used for children whose parents are in prison and for asylum seeking children. When assessing children in need and providing services, specialist assessments may be required and, where possible, should be coordinated so that the child and family experience a coherent process and a single plan of action.

- When undertaking an assessment of a disabled child, the local authority must also consider whether it is necessary to provide support under section 2 of the Chronically Sick and Disabled Persons Act (CSDPA) 1970. Where a local authority is satisfied that the identified services and assistance can be provided under section 2 of the CSDPA, and it is necessary in order to meet a disabled child's needs, it must arrange to provide that support.

- Concerns about maltreatment may be the reason for a referral to local authority children's social care or concerns may arise during the course of providing services to the child and family. In these circumstances, local authority children's social care must initiate enquiries to find out what is happening to the child and whether protective action is required. Local authorities, with the help of other organisations as appropriate, also have a duty to make enquiries under section 47 of the Children Act 1989 if they have reasonable cause to suspect that a child is suffering, or is likely to suffer, significant harm, to enable them to decide whether they should take any action to safeguard and promote the child's welfare. There may be a need for immediate protection whilst the assessment is carried out.

- Some children in need may require accommodation because there is no one who has parental responsibility for them, because they are lost or abandoned or because the person who has been caring for them is prevented from providing them with suitable accommodation or care. Under section 20 of the Children Act 1989, the local authority has a duty to accommodate such children in need in their area.

- Following an application under section 31A, where a child is the subject of a care order, the local authority, as a corporate parent, must assess the child's needs and draw up a care plan which sets out the services which will be provided to meet the child's identified needs.

- If a local authority considers that a young carer [...] may have support needs, they must carry out an assessment under section 17ZA. The local authority must also carry out such an assessment if a young carer, or the parent of a young carer, requests one. Such an assessment must consider whether it is appropriate or excessive for the young carer to provide care for the person in question, in light of the young carer's needs and wishes. The Young Carers' (Needs Assessment) Regulations 2015 require local authorities to look at the needs of the whole family when carrying out a young carers' needs assessment. Young carer's assessments can be combined with assessments of adults in the household, with the agreement of the young carer and adults concerned.

> - If a local authority considers that a parent carer of a disabled child [...] may have support needs, they must carry out an assessment under section 17ZD
> - The local authority must also carry out such an assessment if a parent carer requests one. Such an assessment must consider whether it is appropriate for the parent carer to provide, or continue to provide, care for the disabled child, in light of the parent carer's needs and wishes.
>
> (HM Government, 2015a: pp. 18–19. Crown copyright 2015)

child protection committees. One function of these boards is to undertake serious case reviews (SCRs) and another is to ensure that a review of the death of any child normally resident in the LSCB's area is undertaken by a child death overview panel (CDOP).

Section 58 seeks to clarify that battery cannot be regarded as reasonable punishment.

Section 60 concerns child safety orders (see Chapter 8).

Why might a child be assessed under the Children Act?

Reasons for conducting statutory assessments under the Children Act are helpfully summarised in *Working Together to Safeguard Children* (HM Government, 2015a), and Box 3.1 reproduces that summary. Sections 17ZA and 17ZD in Box 3.1 refer to new provisions relating to young carers and parent carers that have been inserted into Part III of the Children Act 1989 by sections 96 and 97 of the Children and Families Act 2014. These came into force in April 2015.

Conclusion

The Children Act 1989 and the amendments made to it in 2004 cover a number of important topics that professionals in children's mental healthcare need to be familiar with. These include the welfare checklist, how parental responsibility is determined, and aspects of private and public law. It is useful to know when a child or young person might need to be assessed using this legal framework, and the social care responsibilities of local authorities.

CHAPTER 4

Consent to treatment

Historical laws protecting autonomy form the legal basis of consent to treatment in England. Obtaining consent for an intervention has a clinical as well as a legal purpose: to secure cooperation and increase the likelihood of treatment success. It is important to bear in mind that, for those under 16 years of age, emergency treatment that is necessary and cannot be delayed can be given under common law. Medical treatment in an emergency for those aged 16 and above who lack capacity is now governed by the Mental Capacity Act 2005, which has replaced the common law.

When and in what circumstances a child has the capacity to consent to treatment is the central theme of this chapter. It is important for clinicians to know some practical aspects of consent to treatment and understand the scope of parental responsibility when it comes to treating children and young people. It is clinically and historically interesting to know about the seminal Gillick case, the legal principles deriving from it, and the clear distinction that has resulted in law between children of 16 years and above and those who are below 16.

They are these: that with a child under 16 who is not Gillick competent, consent can be given by someone with parental responsibility in accordance with the child's best interests. Yet although a so-called Gillick-competent child under the age of 16 can give consent to an intervention, their refusal can be overruled by someone with parental responsibility or by the court. This can seem confusing, and appears to encapsulate a dilemma not only for the clinician, but also for society. We might wish to recognise adolescent autonomy, but we do not wish that children and young people should be allowed to come to harm on the basis of their own or their parents' refusal of necessary and urgent treatment.

There are, of course, special situations for the giving of consent in cases of mental illness: detention and treatment under the Mental Health Act 1983 is one of these and is discussed in Chapter 6. Consent is not required for treatment of conditions directly resulting from a mental disorder if a child or young person is detained under certain sections of the MHA. An example of this would be feeding for anorexia nervosa in a young person detained under section 3 of the Act. Consent for electroconvulsive therapy (ECT) in the case of a young person is also a special situation discussed in Chapter 6.

There is also some inevitable overlap with the Mental Capacity Act 2005, which applies to young people over 16. Briefly, 16- and 17-year-olds are assumed to have capacity unless it is demonstrated otherwise. This is discussed further in Chapter 7.

However, none of this is straightforward. To try to deal with the topic systematically, I begin this chapter with notes on consent and consent by proxy, after which I consider three areas. The first is the historical background that illuminates apparently confusing lessons from case law. The second concerns professional guidelines and when to involve the court. The third covers the various practical options concerning admission to hospital and treatment for young people with mental disorder, making reference to the two codes of practice: that for the Mental Health Act (Department of Health, 2015) and that for the Mental Capacity Act (Department for Constitutional Affairs, 2007).

What if valid consent is not given?

Any intentional touching of a person without legal justification or consent is a tort (battery), which is essentially unlawful touching. It may also be a crime (assault). In more recent times, a claim of negligence could be made, although several elements need to be present for negligence to be demonstrated (that there is a legal duty of care; that this was breached; that there was direct causation; and that some form of harm resulted: see Jackson, 2013). It is also possible that failure to obtain consent could represent a breach of the patient's rights under Article 3 or 8 of the European Convention on Human Rights (ECHR) (see Chapter 2 above and Gilmore & Herring, 2011: footnote p. 9). Indeed, consent is increasingly a matter of international consensus, and the influence of international law on the Montgomery case (see below) is evident.

What is consent needed for?

Consent is needed for:

▶ medical and nursing procedures
▶ treatment of mental illness
▶ photography, videoing, filming
▶ presence of students for teaching
▶ HIV testing
▶ genetic testing

(Puri *et al*, 2012: p. 132).

What are the forms of consent?

Lawyers are in agreement that the term informed consent (a US term) is misleading, as clearly there is no sharp boundary between informed and uninformed. It has been suggested that the phrase 'sufficiently informed consent' would have served better to reflect the fact that individuals will have different requirements for information, depending on circumstances, expectations and knowledge (Jackson, 2013: p. 168). Jackson also raises important problems with the process of obtaining consent as commonly practised in surgical specialties, for example. The mere act of signing a form fails to acknowledge that the giving of consent may be a continuous process and fails to recognise that consent can be withdrawn at any time. Clinicians are now calling for a different approach in the obtaining of consent (Edozien, 2015).

For consent to be real or valid it must have three aspects:

▶ it is given by a competent person (I discuss the difference between capacity and competence on p. 93)

▶ it is given voluntarily

▶ it is adequately informed

(Kennedy & Grubb, 2000: p. 580).

Consent can be:

▶ implicit: demonstrated, for example, by the patient attending the surgery or holding out an arm for a blood pressure reading; or

▶ explicit: this can be verbal or written.

Note that written consent merely serves as evidence that consent has been obtained (Department of Health, 2009): more important is that the patient acts voluntarily, has been given appropriate information and has capacity to give the consent required (Jackson, 2013: p. 170.) Note also that when a patient consents to a treatment this confers no obligation on the doctor to treat.

What is informed consent?

In the UK until now, the Bolam test has governed how much information should be shared with a patient in order for them to give consent (*Bolam v Friern Hospital Management Committee* [1957]). This test established in case law that 'a doctor was not negligent if he acted in accordance with the practice accepted at the time as proper by a responsible body of medical opinion even though other doctors adopt a different practice' (Kennedy & Grubb, 2000: p. 681).

However, the international trend has been to adopt a standard of what a reasonable patient would want to know: that is to say, a patient-based standard rather than a profession-based one. Various models within this standard are described by Jackson (2013: pp. 184–187), including the reasonable doctor test, the prudent patient test and the subjective standard. The last acknowledges that patients have different needs for information, and seems to reflect the guidance of the General Medical Council (GMC) (2008).

The Montgomery case

In a recent judgment (*Montgomery (Appellant) v Lanarkshire Health Board (Respondent) (Scotland)* [2015]) the matter of how much information to give is fully discussed by the most senior court in the UK. The judgment was made by seven Supreme Court judges, who were all in agreement, and it is worth reading in full. It covers much ground, including the changing nature of the doctor–patient relationship, an acknowledgement that resources available influence treatments offered, and what constitutes risk. In particular, the duty of the doctor to inform patients about risks is discussed. Reference is made to other UK and international case law (in Canada and Australia) that has clearly had a bearing on the judgment, and the GMC guidance is consulted (and, incidentally, holds up well).

When it comes to the continuing application of the Bolam test as described above, the view is quite clear. Especially relevant paragraphs are 86–92, and at 86 the judgment states: 'There is no reason to perpetuate the application of the Bolam test in this context any longer'.

The important principles upheld are several. The clinician will need to present information, and particularly the risks of treatments, to patients in a way that they can understand. In particular, the doctor needs to ensure that the patient is aware of any material risks of the treatment and knows about reasonable alternative treatments (para. 87). Doctors will need to undertake a dialogue with patients in order to achieve this. For clinicians working with children, these conversations may assume a further level of complexity, as those with parental responsibility will often be included in them.

Consent by proxy

One simple way of thinking about consent is that a doctor needs consent from only one source, and there are several possible sources for that consent. It might come from a mature minor, or someone with parental responsibility or the courts. Consent from any of these sources will protect the doctor from criticism.

Generally speaking, if a child lacks capacity to consent to treatment then others with parental responsibility, as defined by the Children Act 1989, must make decisions based on the child's best interests. I have set out the qualifications concerning this in Chapter 3. In particular, consent is required from only one parent, unless serious or controversial medical treatment is being proposed. There may also be a duty for both parents to consult on major life-changing decisions on which they disagree.

The court itself can act as a decision maker by proxy in three ways. These are by wardship, by its inherent jurisdiction and by use of section 8 of the Children Act. Powers within wardship and inherent jurisdiction are unlimited.

▶ Wardship, which enables the court to make decisions about the affairs of minors, derives from an ancient property right. Wardship cannot be used in the case of children who are in care ('looked after children'). If a child is a ward of court, the court must make all important decisions about the child's upbringing.

▶ The inherent jurisdiction of the court derives from a similarly ancient statute by which the mentally incompetent were protected by the Crown under *parens patriae* jurisdiction. This can apply to a single decision, and most usually involves court orders to prevent undesirable association, orders relating to medical treatment and orders to protect abducted children. A novel use of this power to prevent sexual exploitation of the young can be found in *Birmingham City Council v Riaz & Ors (Rev 2)* [2014], at paragraph 44.

▶ Section 8 orders under the Children Act are outlined in Chapter 3, and include prohibited steps orders and specific issue orders, as well as what were known as contact and residence orders, but are now child arrangements orders made by the court (Kennedy & Grubb, 2000).

The scope of parental responsibility

The matter of deciding what is and what is not within the scope of parental responsibility when it comes to decisions and consent about treatments has been somewhat unhelpfully clouded by the term 'zone of parental control'. It appeared briefly in the 2008 Mental Health Act (MHA) Code of Practice for England (Department of Health, 2008), but happily does not recur in the latest version (Department of Health, 2015) (see Chapter 1). As highlighted by Hale (2010: p. 92), although the 2008 code appeared to make reference to case law from Europe in explaining the origin of this concept, in fact it referred only to *Neilsen v Denmark* (1988), a rather extraordinary case in which parental sanction was used to detain a 12-year-old boy on a psychiatric ward for some months.

Incidentally, the European Court of Human Rights in this case found that the boy was not deprived of his liberty, as the hospital admission was considered an appropriate exercise of parental rights. This decision has been called questionable by Mr Justice Munby (as he was then) in *Re A* [2010] and was also thought controversial in the Cheshire West case (see Chapter 1).

The wording of the current MHA Code of Practice is the 'scope of parental responsibility', and although this is not exactly defined (how indeed could it be?) two main indicators are:

▶ Is this is a decision that a parent should reasonably be expected to make?

▶ Are there any factors that might undermine the validity of parental consent?

(Department of Health, 2015: pp. 178–179).

During its fleeting existence, some case law did emerge from attempts to define what was meant by the zone of parental responsibility. One case worth considering is *Re D (A Child: Deprivation of liberty)* [2015], which is discussed in Chapter 2.

Historical background: the Family Law Reform Act, Gillick and the refusal cases

The Family Law Reform Act 1969

Until this legislation was enacted in 1969, there was a lack of clarity about whether young people under the age of majority (then 21) could consent to any treatment without the consent of their parents. The section concerning consent (section 8(1)) is stated thus:

> 'The consent of a minor who has attained the age of sixteen years to any surgical, medical or dental treatment [...] shall be as effective as it would be if he were of full age; and where a minor has by virtue of this section given an effective consent to any treatment it shall not be necessary to obtain any consent for it from his parent or guardian.'

The Mental Capacity Act (MCA) Code of Practice (Department for Constitutional Affairs, 2007: section 12.2) adds that this applies to associated procedures such as investigations, anaesthesia or nursing care, but not to certain other procedures:

> 'It does not apply to some rarer types of procedure (for example, organ donation or other procedures which are not therapeutic for the young person) or research. In those cases, anyone under 18 is presumed to lack legal capacity, subject to the test of 'Gillick competence' (testing whether they are mature and intelligent enough to understand a proposed treatment or procedure).'

The case of Gillick

The Gillick case, now well known for its judgment and for introducing the phrase 'the Gillick-competent child' into the professional lexicon, involved, of course, both consent to treatment and confidentiality. I discuss confidentiality in Chapter 5. It is with consent that we are concerned here.

The case has an interesting history. Moreover, the House of Lords judgment makes compelling reading, not only for the eloquence of the judgments by the five Law Lords, but also for how they signal a change in British social history and the emerging autonomy of girls and young women in the wake of the wider availability of contraceptives.

Incidentally, the term Gillick competence should not be confused with the Fraser guidelines (see Chapter 5 for a discussion of both).

In this context it is helpful to consider how and why this case came about.

Mrs Victoria Gillick objected to the contents of a circular from the Department of Health and Social Security (DHSS) issued in 1974. The circular suggested that contraceptive services should be more available to girls under 16 and that, in some circumstances, doctors could prescribe contraceptives to girls under 16 without the consent of their parents. It should be noted that the wording of the circular, cited in the case, was quite cautious (the quotations in the remainder of this section are taken from *Gillick v West Norfolk and Wisbech Area Health Authority* [1985]):

'"Special care is needed not to undermine parental responsibility and family stability. The Department would therefore hope that in any case where a doctor or other professional worker is approached by a person under the age of 16 for advice in these matters, the doctor, or other professional, will always seek to persuade the child to involve the parent or guardian".'

Mrs Gillick wrote to the area health authority as follows:

'I formally FORBID any medical staff employed by Norfolk A.H.A. to give any contraceptive or abortion advice or treatment whatsoever to my four daughters whilst they are under 16 years without my consent.'

As the health authority would not comply, she brought an action claiming that the advice was wrong and unlawful. She also sought a declaration to this effect.

The case was heard in the High Court in 1984 by Mr Justice Woolf. He rejected the claim and refused to allow the declarations sought by Mrs Gillick. The determined Mrs Gillick, however, appealed and an appeal was allowed. The Court of Appeal reversed the decision by Mr Justice Woolf and agreed with Mrs Gillick. In turn, the DHSS appealed this judgment and this is how the case finally reached the House of Lords to be heard by five Lords: Lords Fraser, Scarman, Bridge, Brandon and Templeman.

In the context of giving his judgment, Lord Fraser said the following:

'parental rights to control a child do not exist for the benefit of the parent. They exist for the benefit of the child and they are justified only in so far as they enable the parent to perform his duties towards the child, and towards other children in the family.'

He also said:

'Once the rule of parents' absolute authority over minor children is abandoned, the solution to the problem in this appeal can no longer be found by referring to rigid parental rights at any particular age. The solution depends on a judgement of what is best for the welfare of the particular child.'

And Lord Scarman added:

'I would hold that as a matter of law the parental right to determine whether or not their minor child below the age of 16 will have medical treatment terminates if and when the child achieves a sufficient understanding and intelligence to enable him or her to understand fully what is proposed. It will be a question of fact whether a child seeking advice has sufficient understanding of what is involved to give a consent valid in law. Until the child achieves the capacity to consent, the parental right to make the decision continues save only in exceptional circumstances.'

But it was a close run thing, as there was not unanimity, and three of the five Lords overruled the appeal and found in favour of the DHSS and against Mrs Gillick, while two did not. The irony is that the actions of a mother who sought to prevent doctors giving contraceptive advice to her daughters (and her campaigning didn't stop with this court judgment) led to her name becoming synonymous with the very thing she was seeking to stop.

Two additional points are worth noting here. The first is that, in 2006, there was an attempt to challenge the principles established by the Gillick case in the light of the Human Rights Act. This was the substance of the Axon case, in which a mother sought to establish her rights under Article 8 of the Human Rights Act, and it is discussed in Chapter 2. The challenge was unsuccessful and the Gillick decision therefore remains robust.

The second is that a subsequent finding has confirmed that Gillick competence applies to the 'staged development of a normal child' and is not lost or acquired on a day-to-day basis (as per Lord Donaldson in *Re R (A Minor) (Wardship: Medical Treatment)* [1991] and discussed in Kennedy & Grubb (2000: p. 635). Compare this with capacity as defined by the Mental Capacity Act (see Chapter 7), which can fluctuate.

From consent to refusal

Following this remarkable case, it was widely understood that a competent child with 'sufficient understanding and intelligence to enable him to understand fully what is proposed' could not only consent to medical treatment but, logically, could also refuse it. However, several cases followed to test this assumption and I will mention two of these heard in the Court of Appeal: *Re R* and *Re W*. The result of these cases (and others that post-dated the Human Rights Act 1998) was that, although a competent child could consent to treatment, the refusal of such a child could be countermanded by someone with parental responsibility.

The refusal cases

Let us first consider *Re R (A Minor) (Wardship: Medical Treatment)* [1991]. This case concerned a young person of almost 16 who presented sometimes with mental disturbance sufficiently severe for her to be thought detainable under the Mental Health Act, but at other times appeared more lucid. There was a complex background of care proceedings. The particular problem for the doctor involved in her care seemed to be that she was not thought to be detainable by an approved social worker under the MHA at a time when she clearly required treatment and was refusing to take it.

Wardship proceedings were initiated by the local authority and the matter for the court to consider was whether treatment could be authorised by the court in the light of R's refusal.

The judge decided to make R, who was by this time under a care order, a ward of court (note that this arrangement would no longer be possible as the Children Act 1989, not then implemented, precludes a child in care being made a ward of court: see Harbour (2008: p. 191). In so doing, the authority of the court was used to sanction medical treatment when R refused it.

Although valid consent for treatment had to be sought somehow (and so the outcome was not in dispute), the legal matter was that Gillick competence was thought not to apply. Why was this?

Doubt was cast on the applicability of *Gillick* to the case by Lord Donaldson's above-mentioned finding that Gillick competence is a developmental concept and that there is no suggestion that it might fluctuate on a day-to-day basis. It was therefore not thought relevant to the case in hand and dismissed as inapplicable.

The other case, *Re W (a minor) (medical treatment)* [1992], concerned a 16-year-old young person with anorexia nervosa. Doctors in charge of her care considered that she needed to be moved to a specialist unit and be fed against her wishes if necessary. The court was therefore asked whether it could authorise such interventions, using its inherent jurisdiction (see p. 41 above). She was at this time under the care of the local authority.

This case, in a similar way to *Re R*, prompted re-examination of the conclusions and applications of the findings from the Gillick case (common law) and from section 8 of the Family Law Reform Act 1969 (statute law).

Although the trial judge, Mr Justice Thorpe, had thought W competent to decide about her treatment, the appeal court (which was again led by Lord Donaldson) was very concerned about the effects of an absolute refusal of treatment in the case of a minor and considered that it had a duty to intervene. The case by then had evolved and the clinical condition of the patient had also clearly deteriorated. Lord Donaldson decided that:

> 'No minor of whatever age has power by refusing consent to treatment to override a consent to treatment by someone who has parental responsibility for the minor and a fortiori consent by the court' (cited in Kennedy & Grubb, 2000: p. 639).

From refusal to controversy

Commentators have subsequently criticised the courts' reasoning in both of these 'provocative' cases (e.g. Kennedy & Grubb, 2000: pp. 984–989; Harbour, 2008: pp. 193–195) on several legal grounds. The judgments have been thought by some to ride roughly over the fundamental respect for autonomy proposed in the Gillick case. Making decisions surely means the ability to agree as well as disagree with what is proposed. Other questions arise concerning the limits of the court's inherent jurisdiction and wardship powers derived from the Crown's historical guardianship over minors (Kennedy & Grubb, 2000: p. 776; Hale & Fortin, 2010: p. 98). More obviously, perhaps a clinician would wonder why the Mental Health Act was not used.

However, there are other views, and the controversy generated by *Re W* and *Re R* is discussed more finely by Gilmore & Herring (2011) in an interesting paper that holds that refusing treatment is not just the opposite of consenting to it. The authors distinguish between two types of refusal: refusal to consent (i.e. to a particular treatment) and refusal of treatment (i.e. to accept any treatment whatsoever), and also expand on the concept of concurrent consent (i.e. powers of consent in both parent and child).

Concurrent consent is present, for example, when a child wishes a parent to consent on the child's behalf.

Gilmore & Herring provide arguments about how it can be ethically defensible that a child has a right to consent to treatment, but does not have a right to refuse the same treatment. These include a consideration of how much risk is involved in the various courses of action. Such an approach, they argue, is quite compatible with human rights legislation, in which there is a need to balance autonomy protected by Article 8 with a child's right to protection from harm, also within that article (see Chapter 2 for more discussion on human rights).

Professional guidelines

There are plenty of guidelines for professionals on consent to treatment in children and young people. The main ones are:

► *0–18 Years: Guidance for all Doctors* (General Medical Council, 2007)

► *Consent: Patients and Doctors Making Decisions Together* (General Medical Council, 2008)

► *Children and Young People Toolkit* (British Medical Association, 2010)

► *Reference Guide to Consent for Examination or Treatment* (Department of Health, 2009)

► *Mental Health Act 1983: Code of Practice* (Department of Health, 2015: Chapter 19).

The guidelines from the GMC and the BMA are especially useful as they cover the four nations (England, Scotland, Wales and Northern Ireland). Together with the Department of Health guidance, they also cover consent for unusual medical procedures such as transplants and research, topics that are beyond the scope of this book.

The guidance in the GMC's *0–18 Years* is quoted in full in Box 4.1. You will note the cautious approach taken in paragraphs 30–33, and also that the standard of understanding as assessed in paragraph 24 is way beyond that required in the Department of Health's *Reference Guide to Consent* (and, others have argued, well beyond that required in an ordinary adult.

The BMA's advice in the *Children and Young People Toolkit* is similar and so will not be discussed further.

Several paragraphs from the *Reference Guide to Consent* raise additional points (Box 4.2). One curious anomaly is the consent to research or blood donation (not covered by the Family Law Reform Act, but possibly covered by the standard of Gillick competence). Other points of note are indications about when court involvement should be sought.

It can be seen that the advice to seek court intervention is given without much hesitation (rather than relying on parental consent); that the concept of sufficient understanding is less stringent than that called

Box 4.1   The GMC's guidance on consent to treatment in children and young people

Assessing the capacity to consent

24   You must decide whether a young person is able to understand the nature, purpose and possible consequences of investigations or treatments you propose, as well as the consequences of not having treatment. Only if they are able to understand, retain, use and weigh this information, and communicate their decision to others can they consent to that investigation or treatment. That means you must make sure that all relevant information has been provided and thoroughly discussed before deciding whether or not a child or young person has the capacity to consent.

25   The capacity to consent depends more on young people's ability to understand and weigh up options than on age. When assessing a young person's capacity to consent, you should bear in mind that:

(a)   at 16 a young person can be presumed to have the capacity to consent (see paragraphs 30 to 33)

(b)   a young person under 16 may have the capacity to consent, depending on their maturity and ability to understand what is involved.

26   It is important that you assess maturity and understanding on an individual basis and with regard to the complexity and importance of the decision to be made. You should remember that a young person who has the capacity to consent to straightforward, relatively risk-free treatment may not necessarily have the capacity to consent to complex treatment involving high risks or serious consequences. The capacity to consent can also be affected by their physical and emotional development and by changes in their health and treatment.

Children and young people who lack the capacity to consent

27   If a child lacks the capacity to consent, you should ask for their parent's consent. It is usually sufficient to have consent from one parent. If parents cannot agree and disputes cannot be resolved informally, you should seek legal advice about whether you should apply to the court.

28   The legal framework for the treatment of 16- and 17-year-olds who lack the capacity to consent differs across the UK:

(a)   In England, Wales and Northern Ireland, parents can consent to investiga-tions and treatment that are in the young person's best interests

(b)   In England and Wales, treatment can also be provided in the young person's best interests without parental consent, although the views of parents may be important in assessing the young person's best interests (see paragraphs 12 and 13)

(c)   In Northern Ireland, treatment can be provided in the young person's best interests if a parent cannot be contacted, although you should seek legal advice about applying for court approval for significant (other than emergency) interventions

(d)   In Scotland, 16- and 17-year-olds who do not have the capacity to consent are treated as adults who lack capacity and treatment may be given to safeguard or promote their health.

Young people who have the capacity to consent

29   You should encourage young people to involve their parents in making important decisions, but you should usually abide by any decision they have the capacity to make themselves (see paragraphs 30 to 33 and paragraphs 46 to 52). You should also consider involving other members of the multi-disciplinary team, an independent advocate or a named or designated doctor for child protection if their involvement would help young people in making decisions.

If a young person refuses treatment

30   Respect for young people's views is important in making decisions about their care. If they refuse treatment, particularly treatment that could save their life or prevent serious deterioration in their health, this presents a challenge that you need to consider carefully.

31   Parents cannot override the competent consent of a young person to treatment that you consider is in their best interests. But you can rely on parental consent when a child lacks the capacity to consent. In Scotland parents cannot authorise treatment a competent young person has refused. In England, Wales and Northern Ireland, the law on parents overriding young people's competent refusal is complex. You should seek legal advice if you think treatment is in the best interests of a competent young person who refuses.

32   You must carefully weigh up the harm to the rights of children and young people of overriding their refusal against the benefits of treatment, so that decisions can be taken in their best interests. In these circumstances, you should consider involving other members of the multi-disciplinary team, an independent advocate, or a named or designated doctor for child protection. Legal advice may be helpful in deciding whether you should apply to the court to resolve disputes about best interests that cannot be resolved informally.

33   You should also consider involving these same colleagues before seeking legal advice if parents refuse treatment that is clearly in the best interests of a child or young person who lacks capacity, or if both a young person with capacity and their parents refuse such treatment.

(General Medical Council, 2007: pp. 11–15)

for by the GMC; and that there is anticipation that the Human Rights Act will be used to challenge the overriding of a competent child's refusal of treatment. However, this does not appear to be the trend and, as mentioned at the beginning of this chapter, there is great reluctance by clinicians, and by the courts, to allow a young person to come to harm because he or she refuses treatment.

The *Glass v United Kingdom* case mentioned in Box 4.2 is unusual in a number of respects. I will not elaborate on it here, save to say that where there are differences in viewpoint, intervention from the court can be helpful in preventing escalating crises.

Box 4.2 Selected paragraphs on treatment consent in young people from the Department of Health's guidance

Young people aged 16–17

4. In order to establish whether a young person aged 16 or 17 has the requisite capacity to consent to the proposed intervention, the same criteria as for adults should be used (see chapter 1, paragraph 2). If a young person lacks capacity to consent because of an impairment of, or a disturbance in the functioning of, the mind or brain then the Mental Capacity Act 2005 will apply in the same way as it does to those who are 18 and over (see chapter 2). If however they are unable to make the decision for some other reason, for example because they are overwhelmed by the implications of the decision, then the Act will not apply to them and the legality of any treatment should be assessed under common law principles. It may be unclear whether a young person lacks capacity within the meaning of the Act. In those circumstances, it would be prudent to seek a declaration from the court. More information on how the Act applies to young people is given in chapter 12 of the Mental Capacity Act (2005) Code of Practice.

Children under 16 – the concept of Gillick competence

5. In the case of *Gillick*, the court held that children who have sufficient understanding and intelligence to enable them to understand fully what is involved in a proposed intervention will also have the capacity to consent to that intervention. This is sometimes described as being 'Gillick competent'. A child of under 16 may be Gillick competent to consent to medical treatment, research, donation or any other activity that requires their consent.

Child or young person with capacity refusing treatment

15. The courts have, in the past, also found that parents can consent to their competent child being treated even where the child/young person is refusing treatment. However, there is no post-Human Rights Act 1998 authority for this proposition, and it would therefore be prudent to obtain a court declaration or decision if faced with a competent child or young person who is refusing to consent to treatment, to determine whether it is lawful to treat the child.

21. The European Court of Human Rights judgment in a case where doctors treated a child contrary to his mother's wishes, without a court order (*Glass v United Kingdom*), made clear that the failure to refer such cases to the court is not only a breach of professional guidance but also potentially a breach of the European Convention on Human Rights. In situations where there is continuing disagreement or conflict between those with parental responsibility and doctors, and where the child is not competent to provide consent, the court should be involved to clarify whether a proposed treatment, or withholding of treatment, is in the child's best interests. Parental refusal can only be overridden in an emergency.'

(Department of Health, 2009: pp. 32, 33, 34, 36)

So, when to involve the court?

Assuming that criteria for detention under the Mental Health Act are not met (see Chapter 6), the court may need to be involved in the following situations.

- For under-16-year-olds:
  - if the child is Gillick competent but refusing treatment, or
  - if the child is not Gillick competent and:
    - ▷ the person with parental responsibility cannot be identified, or
    - ▷ lacks capacity for whatever reason, or
    - ▷ is not acting in best interests of child, or
    - ▷ there is a dispute between those with parental responsibility.
- For 16- and 17-years-olds:
  - if the child has capacity (as defined in the Mental Capacity Act: see Chapter 7) but is refusing treatment
  - if the child does not have capacity and is refusing treatment

(adapted from Richards & Moghul, 2010: p. 145).

What does the MHA Code of Practice say about this matter? It is even less specific:

'In cases where a child or young person cannot be admitted and/or treated informally, and the criteria for detention under the Act are not met, legal advice should be obtained on whether to seek the assistance of the High Court. The court's authorisation may be sought by way of an order or declaration, under its inherent jurisdiction, or for a section 8 order under the Children Act 1989. Whether the court is prepared to assist will depend on the facts of the particular case. It should also be noted that the Court of Protection can make a deprivation of liberty order in respect of young people aged 16 and 17' (Department of Health, 2015: para. 19.52).

A note about consent in controversial treatments and procedures

It would now be unusual to undertake sterilisation to avoid pregnancy, owing to improvements in contraceptive techniques. However, authorisation from the court would be needed if this were the least restrictive alternative (British Medical Association, 2010). Sterilisation for the purpose of medical treatment would not need a court order if supported by two doctors (see *Re E (a minor) (medical treatment)* [1991]), provided that other treatments are not appropriate. See advice from the Department of Health (2009) concerning participation in research and for further sources of advice in cases of bone marrow, blood or organ donation.

Decisions about admission and treatment

Clinicians will have noticed that the very long chapter on children and young people in the MHA Code of Practice (Department of Health, 2015: Chapter 19) is not about the Mental Health Act. This would appear to indicate that this area of mental health law has created a lot of confusion over the question of what legal authority exists to admit a young person to a mental health unit and treat them there. Remember too that the Code applies only to England (as does the National Institute for Mental

Health in England (2009) guidance, which sought to clarify things but obviously doesn't).

The MHA Code of Practice has produced flow diagrams for those who find them helpful (Department of Health, 2015: pp. 198–202), but it notes that these are not actually part of the Code. The table in the publication by South London and Maudsley Foundation Trust (2013: p. 202) is also helpful.

In essence, when deciding whether to admit and treat a young person, the clinician must consider two factors:

▶ whether this is a life-threatening emergency – if it is, then they should treat to save life regardless of the basis for consent

▶ whether or not the young person meets the criteria for detention under the Mental Health Act – if so, an MHA assessment should be arranged (see Chapter 6).

These two considerations trump all other decisions at this stage. If neither holds, then the next decisions are dependent on age and competence.

Under-16-year-olds who are Gillick competent

▶ A Gillick-competent under-16-year-old can be informally admitted to hospital for treatment of a mental disorder if he or she consents.

▶ If the child refuses, treatment could be authorised with parental consent, but the MHA Code of Practice (Department of Health, 2015) considers this unwise (see discussion above). Therefore the intervention of the court should be sought.

Under-16-year-olds who are not Gillick competent

▶ An under-16-year-old who is not Gillick competent can be informally admitted to hospital for treatment of a mental disorder with the consent of someone with parental responsibility, provided that there are no factors undermining the validity of this consent (see above). If there are undermining factors, then intervention of the court should be sought.

16- and 17-year-olds who have capacity to consent

▶ A 16- or 17-year-old can be informally admitted to hospital for treatment of a mental disorder if they have capacity (as defined within the Mental Capacity Act: see Chapter 7) and consent.

▶ If the young person refuses, then intervention of the court should be sought. Section 131 of the Mental Health Act cannot be used for this group (see Chapter 6).

16- and 17-year-olds who do not have capacity to consent

This is more difficult. Although parental responsibility could be used to admit the young person to a treatment unit, there are two problems with

51

this. First, it is questionable whether this falls within the usual realm of parenting decisions, or at least as they are set out in the MHA Code of Practice (Department of Health, 2015: para. 19.41). How often is an event of this kind part of what an ordinary parent does?

Second, it is also questionable whether using the Mental Capacity Act (see Chapter 7) is appropriate for other aspects of admission and treatment. Although the MCA Code of Practice (Department for Constitutional Affairs, 2007: para. 12.21) suggests that it is possible to admit a young person who lacks capacity (as defined under the Act) using parental consent, the Act does not allow any actions that result in a deprivation of liberty. In-patient units are structured in such a way that free entry and exit are carefully monitored (necessarily, to safeguard the residents) and this is very likely to raise the matter of whether this constitutes a deprivation of liberty according to ECHR provisions. In addition, there are restrictions on the management of challenging behaviour and the use of restraint under the MCA (see Chapter 7).

For all these reasons, use of the MCA to admit a young person to an in-patient unit is problematic, and if he or she does not meet the criteria for detention under the MHA, the clinician would be well advised to seek the intervention of the court. A comparison of the use of the MHA and the MCA is made in Chapter 7.

This is all somewhat bewildering for clinicians. As summarised by Barber *et al* (2012), if the Codes of Practice are being followed, these changes in the law seem likely to increase either the number of detentions under the MHA, or the number of requests to the courts for intervention or both.

Conclusion

It is important for clinicians to be aware that the gaining of consent is a process requiring some consideration. This has been highlighted in the Montgomery case, which emphasised the duty of the doctor to ensure that the patient is aware of any material risks associated with a treatment and also knows about reasonable alternative treatments. For CAMHS clinicians, these conversations will often include those with parental responsibility. The rest of this chapter has given a historical perspective to consent and refusal, and outlined key information from professional guidelines. Finally, the notes on decision-making about admission and treatment provide guidance on dealing with some clinical situations, but do not offer all the answers. In particular, the tension surrounding the admission of children and young people who refuse it is a major difficulty as the law currently stands. Clinicians are understandably reluctant to use the Mental Health Act, and professional guidance tends to recommend the seeking of legal advice, which is costly and time-consuming.

This is an unhelpful situation for both patients and clinicians.

CHAPTER 5

Confidentiality

Confidentiality has been a cornerstone of British medical practice for decades and traditionally has been governed by common law. That patients can trust doctors is essential to making diagnoses and suggesting treatments, and the general rule has been that information relating to patients has been disclosed only with the patient's consent. Broadly, in this respect, children and young people have the same entitlement to confidentiality as adults.

However, maintaining patients' confidentiality, whether they are adults or children, has never been an absolute duty, and information can be disclosed without a patient's consent by law or in the public interest (discussed below), particularly when child protection is involved.

In law, doctors have an obligation to disclose information when ordered to do so by a judge or a court of law in both civil and criminal proceedings, and this includes the coroner's court. The guidance issued by the General Medical Council (GMC; 2009) gives useful information about this. Doctors can also, of course, be summoned to give evidence and can be held in contempt of court if they fail to attend.

In fact, a surprising number of regulatory bodies and statutes provide for some form of access to otherwise confidential information. These are discussed in the GMC guidance, and they cover, for example, the handling of information about certain notifiable diseases.

It may also be relevant to know briefly about two recent pieces of statute law that might affect confidentiality: these are the National Health Service Act 2006 and the Serious Crimes Act 2015.

The National Health Service Act 2006 introduced a provision (in section 251) that enables the common law duty of confidentiality to be overridden. This means that confidential patient information can be disclosed for medical purposes where it is not possible to use anonymised information and where seeking consent is not practical. The NHS Health Research Authority has established a Confidentiality Advisory Group to deal with this new function (Health Research Authority, 2015).

This piece of legislation serves to emphasise the connections between confidentiality, medical records and information governance, which is becoming an increasingly complex area. In relation to this, clinicians should be aware that each NHS organisation should have a Caldicott guardian. This is usually a senior person responsible for ensuring the confidentiality of patient information (for a description of this role see Roch-Bery, 2003).

Another and more recent piece of legislation having a bearing on confidentiality is the Serious Crimes Act 2015. A duty is now imposed as part of this Act to notify the chief officer of police if an act of female genital mutilation appears to have been carried out on a girl under 18 years of age. Clinicians need to know this if their case-load includes those at risk of this practice.

On a more day-to-day level, the other statutes that are relevant to confidentiality and children's mental health law are the Human Rights Act 1998 and the Data Protection Act 1998. Clinicians need to be aware of the guidance from professional organisations, principally the GMC (2007, 2009), but also the Department of Health and the British Medical Association (BMA). Two cases of particular relevance to confidentiality, the Gillick and Axon cases, already introduced in earlier chapters, will be revisited for what they can tell us about this topic. The guidance *Working Together to Safeguard Children* (HM Government, 2015a) has a great deal to say on the matter of sharing information that would ordinarily be confidential, and this will be mentioned, along with some detail on what constitutes a disclosure in the public interest. Finally, guidelines on who can access clinical information will be briefly described.

Note that the Freedom of Information Act 2000 does not cover personal information.

First, what is meant by confidential patient information?

The Department of Health (2003: para. 9, p. 7) describes confidential patient information as follows:

> 'A duty of confidence arises when one person discloses information to another (e.g. patient to clinician) in circumstances where it is reasonable to expect that the information will be held in confidence. It –
>
> a. is a legal obligation that is derived from case law;
> b. is a requirement established within professional codes of conduct; and
> c. must be included within NHS employment contracts as a specific requirement linked to disciplinary procedures.'

The Human Rights Act 1998

The relevant article in the Human Rights Act (and in the European Convention on Human Rights (ECHR)) is Article 8: the right to respect for private and family life (Box 5.1) (see also Chapter 2).

A key principle from ECHR legislation is proportionality, so in the matter of confidentiality, a balance needs to be met between the rights of the child or young person and the interests of the community. There will

---

Box 5.1 Article 8 of the Human Rights Act

Right to respect for private and family life

1. Everyone has the right to respect for his private and family life, his home and his correspondence.
2. There shall be no interference by a public authority with the exercise of this right except such as is in accordance with the law and is necessary in a democratic society in the interests of national security, public safety or the economic well-being of the country, for the prevention of disorder or crime, for the protection of health or morals, or for the protection of the rights and freedoms of others.

---

also need to be a balance between competing Convention rights. This is demonstrated in the Axon case, which is discussed in Chapter 2 and is referred to below.

The Data Protection Act

The eight principles of the Data Protection Act 1998 are described in Schedule 1 of the Act. For example, the third principle is that personal data should be 'adequate, relevant, and not excessive' and the fifth that data 'shall not be kept for longer than is necessary for that purpose'. Data can be shared without consent only where this is 'necessary'. At the time of writing, a new European Data Protection Regulation was due for publication by the European Union in May 2016 and intended to apply from May 2018. It seems likely to include terms of ownership of data and a right that data be forgotten. However, it is unclear yet how this will affect the use of healthcare data in the UK.

For the purposes of the Data Protection Act, processing (i.e what one does with data) includes holding, disclosing or obtaining personal data, and the data include all forms of media, including images as well as documents (Department of Health, 2003). The Act applies to living individuals of all ages.

What does the GMC say about confidentiality and young people?

The following paragraphs of *0–18 Years: Guidance for all Doctors* (General Medical Council, 2007: pp. 18, 19) are especially relevant:

> '43   The same duties of confidentiality apply when using, sharing or disclosing information about children and young people as about adults. You should:
>
> a   disclose information that identifies the patient only if this is necessary to achieve the purpose of the disclosure – in all other cases you should anonymise the information before disclosing it

    b   inform the patient* about the possible uses of their information, including how it could be used to provide their care and for clinical audit

    c   ask for the patient's consent before disclosing information that could identify them, if the information is needed for any other purpose, other than in the exceptional circumstances described in this guidance

    d   keep disclosures to the minimum necessary.

*or, where appropriate, those with parental responsibility for the patient.

46   If a child or young person does not agree to disclosure there are still circumstances in which you should disclose information:

    a   when there is an overriding public interest in the disclosure

    b   when you judge that the disclosure is in the best interests of a child or young person who does not have the maturity or understanding to make a decision about disclosure

    c   when disclosure is required by law.'

And the Department of Health?

From Department of Health (2003: para. 9, p. 30):

'Young people aged 16 or 17 are presumed to be competent for the purposes of consent to treatment and are therefore entitled to the same duty of confidentiality as adults. Children under the age of 16 who have the capacity and understanding to take decisions about their own treatment are also entitled to make decisions about the use and disclosure of information they have provided in confidence (e.g. they may be receiving treatment or counselling about which they do not want their parents to know).'

This reflects the Gillick case (see below). For the connection with treatment decisions this paragraph continues:

'However, where a competent young person or child is refusing treatment for a life threatening condition, the duty of care would require confidentiality to be breached to the extent of informing those with parental responsibility for the child who might then be able to provide the necessary consent to the treatment.'

Confidentiality in *Gillick* and *Axon*

The Gillick case, described in Chapter 4, involved both consent to treatment and confidentiality. The two are necessarily entwined: it would be impossible for a parent or someone with parental responsibility to give consent by proxy without knowledge of what the consent was being sought for. It is with confidentiality that we are concerned here.

As described in Chapter 4, Mrs Victoria Gillick objected to the contents of a circular from the Department of Health and Social Security (DHSS) which suggested that, in some exceptional circumstances, doctors could prescribe contraceptives to girls under the age of 16 without consulting their parents.

The case was heard in the High Court in 1984 by Mr Justice Woolf. He rejected the claim, an appeal was allowed, and the Court of Appeal reversed the decision. In turn, the DHSS appealed this judgment and the case finally reached the House of Lords.

In addition to the extracts from the judgment already quoted in Chapter 4, some additional comments of Lord Fraser are worth citing. In the context of his speech about giving contraceptive advice to girls under the age of 16 he said:

'But there may well be cases, and I think there will be some cases, where the girl refuses either to tell the parents herself or to permit the doctor to do so and in such cases the doctor will, in my opinion, be justified in proceeding without the parents' consent or even knowledge provided he is satisfied on the following matters:

(1)   that the girl (although under 16 years of age) will understand his advice

(2)   that he cannot persuade her to inform her parents or to allow him to inform the parents that she is seeking contraceptive advice

(3)   that she is very likely to begin or to continue having sexual intercourse with or without contraceptive treatment

(4)   that unless she receives contraceptive advice or treatment her physical or mental health or both are likely to suffer

(5)   that her best interests require him to give her contraceptive advice, treatment or both without the parental consent'

(*Gillick v West Norfolk and Wisbech Area Health Authority* [1985]).

These five points have become known as the Fraser guidelines.

Incidentally, there has been some confusion about the terms Gillick competence and the Fraser guidelines, with some people using them interchangeably. This has been the subject of an editorial in the *British Medical Journal* (Wheeler, 2006). The so-called Fraser guidelines, given as part of the judgment, are specific to the giving of contraceptives. Gillick competence, on the other hand, has now embraced a wider meaning. These terms should be kept distinct.

The case of Axon some years later, in 2006, centrally concerned how medical professionals should deal with young people who want advice on sexual matters, but who cannot be persuaded to inform their parents or to allow the medical professional to inform them. In relation to advice issued by the Department of Health in 2004, Mrs Axon sought:

'1.   A declaration that the 2004 Guidance is unlawful in that it:

(1)   misrepresents the decision of the House of Lords in Gillick whilst purporting to clarify it;

(2)   makes doctors and other health professionals the sole arbiters of what is in the best interests of a child;

(3)   makes informing parents the exception rather than the rule;

(4) excludes parents from important decision-making about the life and welfare of their child;

(5) fails in any event to discharge the State's positive obligation to give practical and effective protection to the Claimant's rights under article 8(1).

2. A declaration that, other than in circumstances where disclosure would be likely to damage the child's physical or mental health:

(1) doctors and other health professionals have a duty to consult the parents of a young person under 16 before providing advice and/ or treatment in respect of contraception, sexually transmitted infections or abortions;

(2) parents have a right to be informed about the proposed provision of advice and/or treatment in respect of contraception, sexually transmitted infections or abortions'

(R (on the application of Axon) v Secretary of State for Health [2006]).

So in going further than merely challenging the Gillick case and the advice of the Department of Health, she also considered that her ECHR Article 8 rights were not being protected.

In reviewing the details of the speeches made in the House of Lords judgments on the Gillick case by Lords Scarman and Fraser, the presiding judge, Mr Justice Silber, emphasised:

'It is noteworthy that both Lord Fraser and Lord Scarman sanctioned the provision of advice and treatment to young persons on sexual matters not only without parental consent but also without parental knowledge.'

As part of his judgment, which upholds the lawfulness of the Department of Health guidelines and the Gillick principle, he gives several reasons for not allowing that the Department of Health guidance interferes with any Article 8 rights of a parent, including that: 'it is established that a child's article 8 rights override similar rights of a parent'. In other words the interests of the child predominate.

And so the judgment at paragraph 154 upheld these principles:

'(1) that the young person although under 16 years of age understands all aspects of the advice [In the light of Lord Scarman's comments in Gillick [...] he or she must 'have sufficient maturity to understand what is involved': that understanding includes all relevant matters and it is not limited to family and moral aspects as well as all possible adverse consequences which might follow from the advice];

(2) that the medical professional cannot persuade the young person to inform his or her parents or to allow the medical professional to inform the parents that their child is seeking advice and/or treatment on sexual matters [As stated in the 2004 Guidance, where the young person cannot be persuaded to involve a parent, every effort should be made to persuade the young person to help find another adult (such as another family member or a specialist youth worker) to provide support to the young person];

(3) that […] the young person is very likely to begin or to continue having sexual intercourse with or without contraceptive treatment or treatment for a sexually transmissible illness;

(4) that unless the young person receives advice and treatment on the relevant sexual matters, his or her physical or mental health or both are likely to suffer […] and

(5) that the best interests of the young person require him or her to receive advice and treatment on sexual matters without parental consent or notification'

(R (on the application of Axon) v Secretary of State for Health [2006]).

Disclosing confidential information

Practitioners frequently face difficulties in knowing whether to breach confidentiality in a doctor–patient relationship with a child or young person. As described by Harbour (2008), there is actually no basis in law for the frequently held assumption that disclosing confidential information is in the best interests of the child. However, the findings of serious case reviews have persistently encouraged information sharing. *Working Together to Safeguard Children* (HM Government, 2015a: pp. 16–17), in particular, states:

'23. Early sharing of information is the key to providing effective early help where there are emerging problems […]. Serious Case Reviews (SCRs) have shown how poor information sharing has contributed to the deaths or serious injuries of children.

24. Fears about sharing information cannot be allowed to stand in the way of the need to promote the welfare and protect the safety of children.'

To emphasise the point and encourage professionals not to allow the Data Protection Act and Human Rights Act to serve as barriers to information sharing, the government issued *Information Sharing: Advice for Practitioners Providing Safeguarding Services to Children, Young People, Parents and Carers* (HM Government, 2015b). It lists 'seven golden rules to sharing information', which can be summarised as follows: the sharing of any personal information must be necessary, proportionate and relevant, and the information shared should be adequate, accurate, timely and secure.

As will be seen, there is variability in what is seen as good practice, and, as interpretations could differ, the clinician has to exercise careful judgement in each case.

What exactly is meant by disclosures in the public interest?

It is a fortunate fact that doctors, unlike judges, do not have to make decisions about disclosing information that the media can then make public. Although there can be strong grounds for public debate about important aspects of the care of very unwell infants, for example, there can also be compelling reasons to maintain confidentiality not only to protect the child at the centre of proceedings, but also to shield those with parental responsibility, carers and hospital staff from consequent pressures. These arguments were marshalled in *Re C (A Minor) (Wardship: Medical Treatment) (No. 2)* [1990], which concerned a seriously ill baby who was a ward of court and in whom a national newspaper took great interest. An order was made to prevent disclosure of any information that could lead to the identification of the child.

Far more likely for doctors are considerations of whether harm is likely to arise to their child patient.

From the GMC again (2007: p. 21):

'49   [...] you should disclose information if this is necessary to protect the child or young person, or someone else, from risk of death or serious harm. Such cases may arise, for example, if:

a   a child or young person is at risk of neglect or sexual, physical or emotional abuse [...]

b   the information would help in the prevention, detection or prosecution of serious crime, usually crime against the person

c   a child or young person is involved in behaviour that might put them or others at risk of serious harm, such as serious addiction, self-harm or joy-riding.'

And regarding disclosures when a child lacks the capacity to consent (General Medical Council, 2007: p. 22):

'51   Children will usually be accompanied by parents or other adults involved in their care and you can usually tell if a child agrees to information being shared by their behaviour. Occasionally, children who lack the capacity to consent will share information with you on the understanding that their parents are not informed. You should usually try to persuade the child to involve a parent in such circumstances. If they refuse and you consider it is necessary in the child's best interests for the information to be shared (for example, to enable a parent to make an important decision, or to provide proper care for the child), you can disclose information to parents or appropriate authorities. You should record your discussions and reasons for sharing the information.'

The guidance from the Department of Health (2003, p. 34) is wider. On the subject of common law and disclosure in the public interest, this states:

'30.   Under common law, staff are permitted to disclose personal information in order to prevent and support detection, investigation and punishment of serious crime and/or to prevent abuse or serious harm to others where they judge, on a case by case basis, that the public good that would be achieved by the disclosure outweighs both the obligation of confidentiality to the individual patient concerned and the broader public interest in the provision of a confidential service.

31.   Whoever authorises disclosure must make a record of any such circumstances, so that there is clear evidence of the reasoning used

and the circumstances prevailing. Disclosures in the public interest should also be proportionate and be limited to relevant details. It may be necessary to justify such disclosures to the courts or to regulatory bodies and a clear record of the decision making process and the advice sought is in the interest of both staff and the organisations they work within.

32. Wherever possible the issue of disclosure should be discussed with the individual concerned and consent sought. Where this is not forthcoming, the individual should be told of any decision to disclose against his/her wishes. This will not be possible in certain circumstances, e.g. where the likelihood of a violent response is significant or where informing a potential suspect in a criminal investigation might allow them to evade custody, destroy evidence or disrupt an investigation.

33. Each case must be considered on its merits. Decisions will sometimes be finely balanced and staff may find it difficult to make a judgement. It may be necessary to seek legal or other specialist advice from professional, regulatory or indemnifying bodies) or to await or seek a court order. Staff need to know who and where to turn to for advice in such circumstances.'

Box 5.2 reproduces examples that the guidance gives of disclosure to protect the public.

Box 5.2 Examples of disclosure to protect the public

Serious Crime and National Security

The definition of serious crime is not entirely clear. Murder, manslaughter, rape, treason, kidnapping, child abuse or other cases where individuals have suffered serious harm may all warrant breaching confidentiality. Serious harm to the security of the state or to public order and crimes that involve substantial financial gain or loss will also generally fall within this category. In contrast, theft, fraud or damage to property where loss or damage is less substantial would generally not warrant breach of confidence.

Risk of Harm

Disclosures to prevent serious harm or abuse also warrant breach of confidence. The risk of child abuse or neglect, assault, a traffic accident or the spread of an infectious disease are perhaps the most common that staff may face. However, consideration of harm should also inform decisions about disclosure in relation to crime. Serious fraud or theft involving NHS resources would be likely to harm individuals waiting for treatment. A comparatively minor prescription fraud may actually be linked to serious harm if prescriptions for controlled drugs are being forged. It is also important to consider the impact of harm or neglect from the point of view of the victim(s) and to take account of psychological as well as physical damage. For example, the psychological impact of child abuse or neglect may harm siblings who know of it in addition to the child concerned.

(Department of Health, 2003: p. 35)

And finally for the record: access to health information about young people

Since the Access to Health Records Act 1990, all patients have had a right to gain access to their health records. A fairly frequent problem for clinicians is requests for access to clinical notes about young people. Not only can competent children (in the sense of Gillick competent) request such access, but they can also authorise others to do so on their behalf. The BMA (2010: pp. 28–32) gives full guidance on access, and specifically on competence to consent to disclosure:

> 'In England, Wales and Northern Ireland children who are aged 12 or over are generally expected to have competence to give or withhold their consent to the release of information. In Scotland, anyone aged 12 or over is legally presumed to have such competence' (p. 28).

The guidance adds that younger children may also be able to make decisions about their own health information if they are competent to do so and, unless there are good reasons to suggest otherwise (for example, if abuse is suspected), health professionals should respect their wishes that parents or guardians should not know all or some aspects of their healthcare. So, children and young people who are competent can apply to see their health records, as can anyone with parental responsibility (see below). However, both the BMA (p. 32) and the GMC (2007, p. 23) stipulate that, if access to information is likely to cause serious harm or divulge information about another person without that person's consent, then they should not have access.

Concerning parents who want access

It should be noted that the person with parental responsibility is not necessarily the same as the nearest relative. The term nearest relative has particular meaning in the Mental Health Act, and this role is discussed further in Chapter 6.

In the case of parents, the BMA (2010: p. 31) states:

> 'Anyone with parental responsibility has a statutory right to apply for access to their child's health records. If the child is capable of giving consent, access may only be given with his or her consent. It may be necessary to discuss parental access alone with children if there is a suspicion that they are under pressure to agree. (For example, the young person may not wish a parent to know about a request for contraceptive advice.) If a child lacks the competence to understand the nature of an application but access would be in his or her best interests, it should be granted. Parental access must not be given where it conflicts with the child's best interests and any information that a child revealed in the expectation that it would not be disclosed should not be released unless it is in the child's best interests to do so. Where parents are separated and one of them applies for access to the medical record, doctors are under no obligation to inform the other parent, although they may consider doing so if they believe it to be in the child's best interests.'

In spite of guidelines and the law, we know that doctors will display a variation of behaviours and attitudes towards patient confidentiality and the involvement of relatives in patient care (see for example Gilbar, 2012). The management of challenging mental health problems in children and young people has always required a careful and diplomatic approach.

In practice, it seems likely that in disputes about confidentiality involving children or young people (and adults who lack capacity) there will be a balancing by the court of common law, the Data Protection Act and the Human Rights Act.

Although not concerning a young person, as part of the judgment made by Mrs Justice Hale in R *(on the application of Stevens) v Plymouth City Council & Anor* [2002] this tension is acknowledged:

'32.   The simple answer to this case is that, both at common law and under the Human Rights Act, a balance must be struck between the public and private interests in maintaining the confidentiality of this information and the public and private interests in permitting, indeed requiring, its disclosure for certain purposes. [...]

33.   The common law obligation to keep a confidence is conceptually quite different from the statutory obligation to process data in accordance with the data protection principles and from the right to respect for private life enshrined in Article 8(1) of the European Convention on Human Rights, although there are overlaps. [...]

34.   Even where information is covered by an obligation of confidence, the breadth of that obligation depends upon the circumstances [...]. If the information has been brought into existence for certain authorised purposes, then it can be disclosed for those purposes. Thus, for example, the medical reports and recommendations have to be disclosed to the applicant approved social worker and to the local authority in order for them to fulfil their statutory functions. It would scarcely be a large step to include the nearest relative within that loop.'

Conclusion

There are thus many limits to confidentiality in the doctor–patient relationship with a child or young person. Clinicians need to be aware of the professional guidelines on confidentiality and who can access clinical information and also of the seemingly broadening definitions of what is meant by the public interest.

The statutes that are of particular relevance to confidentiality and children's mental health law are the Human Rights Act 1998 and the Data Protection Act 1998. Much guidance is also available from the GMC, Department of Health and BMA.

The two cases of particular relevance to confidentiality, the Gillick and Axon cases, inform us about case law and a Human Rights Act challenge to it. The guidance *Working Together to Safeguard Children* (HM Government, 2015a) has a great deal to say on the matter of sharing information that would ordinarily be confidential.

CHAPTER 6

The Mental Health Act

The Mental Health Act 1983 (MHA) covers the reception, care and treatment of mentally disordered persons in England and Wales. For practical purposes, it is the legislation used when patients are admitted to, detained and treated in hospital without their consent. Using this legislation will be a familiar task to child and adolescent psychiatrists, even if an uncommon one. The politics and use of resources involved in the use of the Act are, however, sometimes fraught and complex. This is because, at the very least, detaining a young person requires a tier 4 bed, and although these have never been easy to find, it has now become very difficult. There has also been national concern in the past few years about the use of police cells in detaining children and young people on section 136 of the Act (see below).

The parliamentary debates on these subjects are interesting to follow. The reasons for the shortage of beds undoubtedly include increased demand and decreased capacity of local authority social care services and community CAMHS to deal with it, associated with changes in commissioning arrangements that make everything more complex. In England, NHS England took over commissioning of tier 4 in-patient services in April 2013. The House of Commons Health Select Committee has been critical of NHS England and the fact that it has failed to develop systems to manage the problem (Health Select Committee, 2014: Recommendations 11 and 12). Although further discussion of this is beyond the scope of this book, clinicians are uneasy about the practice of placing adolescents in in-patient beds often at great distance from their family homes. Surely, one would have thought, this must engage a young person's Article 8 right to family life.

Since the introduction of the Health and Social Care Act 2008, the Care Quality Commission (CQC) has had a specific responsibility for reviewing the use of the MHA in England. This includes inspecting, regulating and monitoring places where people are detained. The CQC also has a duty to appoint second opinion appointed doctors (SOADs) (Department of Health, 2015). The way this is done is constantly changing, and since April 2014 an MHA reviewer has been included in the inspection team. These were functions previously undertaken by the Mental Health Act Commission (MHAC), which operated in England and Wales and was abolished in 2009.

The MHAC had been concerned about the number of children and young people detained on adult psychiatric wards and collected data to this end. To give an idea of how many individuals this applied to, Harbour (2008: p. 77) notes that 310 children and adolescents were detained and resident on adult wards within the public and private healthcare estate on 31 March 2007.

The amendments to the MHA 1983 introduced by the 2007 amendment Act appeared to address this concern, and made it a new duty for hospital managers to ensure that anyone under the age of 18 is admitted, formally or informally, to an age-appropriate environment. Other changes brought in by the 2007 amendments are summarised later in this chapter.

From December 2008, the admission to an adult psychiatric ward of any child under the age of 16 has constituted a serious untoward incident (Puri *et al*, 2012: p. 198). According to the new MHA Code of Practice (Department of Health, 2015: para 19.93), the CQC must be informed if a young person under the age of 18 remains longer than 48 hours on an adult psychiatric ward.

Although the numbers of children and young people detained under the MHA are thought to be low (with one source giving a number of 350 a year, according to Pugh, 2008), I have found it surprisingly difficult to obtain any data relating to the use of the Act for this age group. NHS England does not collect data on detained patients. The CQC does not collect data on children detained under the MHA now either, but it has been collecting data since April 2013 on notifications received of children admitted to adult psychiatric wards. Between 2006 and 2009, when the CQC did collect data for England on individuals under the age of 18 detained in CAMHS facilities, figures climbed steadily, from 294 to 381 (Care Quality Commission, 2010).

The Health and Social Care Information Centre (HSCIC) does have some data on children and young people detained under the MHA in specialist adult mental health services (but not including CAMHS, learning disability services or acute hospitals, making the figures of little value in indicating the total number detained under the Act). These figures, from the Mental Health Minimum Data Set (MHMDS) 2013–2014 list for England and Wales show that there were 47 detentions on adult wards for males under 18 years of age and 56 for females (Health and Social Care Information Centre, 2014).

Thus, it is highly likely that the practice of detaining children and young people on adult wards continues, and this is hardly surprising when the bed situation is so dire. Of course, it may be appropriate in some circumstances, such as when the 18th birthday is very near and the provision is close to home or the patient prefers it. Furthermore, it can be a traumatic experience for a young person to be admitted to an age-appropriate bed several hundred miles away after a delay of several days: a situation that is currently common, risky and unacceptable.

There is no lower age limit for use of the MHA, including the imposition of community treatment orders. Thomas *et al* (2015) describe using section 2 of the Act with an 8-year-old. Interestingly, Lady Hale has noted a reluctance among clinicians to use the Act, although according to this senior judge, 'there is much to be said [for using it] from the child's point of view' (Hale, 2010: p. 91).

What are the main amendments of the MHA 2007 specific to children and young people?

► The definition of mental disorder is broadened.

► Approved mental health professionals (AMHPs) replace approved social workers (ASWs), and responsible clinicians (RCs) replace responsible medical officers (RMOs).

► Capacitous 16- and 17-year-olds can both consent to or refuse admission, and this may not be overruled by those with parental authority (section 131).

► The treatability test has been replaced with an appropriate medical treatment test (for sections 3 and 37).

► Extra safeguards are introduced concerning electroconvulsive therapy (ECT): except in an emergency, ECT for under-18s must always be approved by a second opinion approved doctor, even if they consent (section 58A).

► All detained under-18s must be referred annually to a mental health tribunal (still known in Wales as a mental health review tribunal) whether or not they request a tribunal hearing (section 68).

► Hospital managers have a duty to ensure that under-18s, both detained and voluntary patients, are accommodated in an environment that is suitable for their age (subject to need); they must consult with a suitable specialist to determine the appropriateness of the environment (section 131A).

► There are restrictions to the informal admission of 16- and 17-year-olds. If a young person of this age group (who has capacity) does not consent to admission, then no one with parental responsibility can consent to it either.

(The above list is adapted from Barber *et al*, 2012: pp. 5–7.)

Consent to admission and parental responsibility are discussed in Chapter 4. In the remainder of this chapter, I will consider three broad areas: first, the principles of the MHA, the process of detaining a person and the people involved in this process; second, treatments; and third, the MHA in practice. For brevity, aspects of the Act (such as the appeals procedure and applications to mental health tribunals) are not covered if they are discussed elsewhere or are not specific to children and young people.

Principles, process and people

Principles

A note on the Code of Practice

It should be noted that there are two MHA Codes of Practice: one for England and one for Wales. In this book the code referred to is the one for England (Department of Health, 2015), Chapter 19 of which deals with children and young people.

Readers of the Code of Practice and of the MHA itself will notice some difference in emphasis between them. In particular, the Code is extremely detailed in some parts, for example concerning decision-making or when it might or might not be appropriate to admit a young person to an adult bed, whereas the Act is concise. This probably reflects the fact that the MHA is not really focused on the needs of children and young people and also how complex the legislation surrounding mental health law for this age group has become.

The Code, written by the Secretary of State as required by the MHA, provides guidance to registered medical practitioners (doctors), approved clinicians, managers and staff of hospitals, and approved mental health professionals on how to administer the Act. Although not legally binding, there is an expectation that, if professionals depart from its guidance, they give a reason for doing so.

It is worth listing the overall guiding principles of the Code before looking at the specific principles for children and young people. The five guiding principles for the Code as a whole are:

▶ using the least restrictive option
▶ empowerment and involvement
▶ respect and dignity
▶ purpose and effectiveness
▶ efficiency and equity.

The influence of the first of these is strong in clinicians' minds and there has probably been a reluctance to use the MHA if it can be avoided. Perhaps, however, this reluctance needs to be questioned in the light of the difficulties in using alternative legislation, such as the Mental Capacity Act (see Chapter 7) and, to a limited extent, the Children Act (see Chapter 3).

Box 6.1 shows some of the general considerations specific to children and young people given in the Code.

Definition of mental disorder

Following the 2007 amendments to the MHA, section 1(2) of the Act now defines mental disorder as any disorder or disability of the mind. The previously existing categories of mental disorder (mental illness, mental impairment, severe mental impairment and psychopathic disorder) have

---

Box 6.1 Mental Health Act Code of Practice for England: some considerations specific to children and young people under the age of 18

When making decisions in relation to the care and treatment of children and young people, practitioners should keep the following points in mind:

- the best interests of the child or young person must always be a significant consideration
- everyone who works with children has a responsibility for keeping them safe and to take prompt action if welfare needs or safeguarding concerns are identified
- all practitioners and agencies are expected to contribute to whatever actions are needed to safeguard and promote a child or young person's welfare
- the developmental process from childhood to adulthood, particularly during adolescence, involves significant changes in a wide range of areas, such as physical, emotional and cognitive development – these factors need to be taken into account, in addition to the child and young person's personal circumstances, when assessing whether a child or young person has a mental disorder
- children and young people should always be kept as fully informed as possible and should receive clear and detailed information concerning their care and treatment, explained in a way they can understand and in a format that is appropriate to their age
- the child or young person's views, wishes and feelings should always be sought, their views taken seriously and professionals should work with them collaboratively in deciding on how to support that child or young person's needs
- any intervention in the life of a child or young person that is considered necessary by reason of their mental disorder should be the least restrictive option and the least likely to expose them to the risk of any stigmatisation, consistent with effective care and treatment, and it should also result in the least possible separation from family, carers, friends and community or interruption of their education
- where hospital admission is necessary, the child or young person should be placed as near to their home as reasonably practicable, recognising that placement further away from home increases the separation between the child or young person and their family, carers, friends, community and school
- all children and young people should receive the same access to educational provision as their peers
- children and young people have as much right to expect their dignity to be respected as anyone else, and
- children and young people have as much right to privacy and confidentiality as anyone else

(Department of Health, 2015: para. 19.5, p. 169)

---

disappeared. This broader definition of mental disorder effectively means that any childhood psychiatric disorder could now fall within its definition.

Examples of clinically recognised mental disorders from the Code of Practice (Department of Health, 2015: p. 26) include, but are not confined to:

▶ affective disorders such as depression and bipolar disorder

▶ schizophrenia and delusional disorders

- neurotic, stress-related and somatoform disorders, such as anxiety, phobic disorders, obsessive–compulsive disorders, post-traumatic stress disorder and hypochondriacal disorders
- organic mental disorders such as dementia and delirium (however caused)
- personality and behavioural changes caused by brain injury or damage (however acquired)
- personality disorders
- mental and behavioural disorders caused by psychoactive substance use
- eating disorders, non-organic sleep disorders and non-organic sexual disorders
- learning (intellectual) disability (see below)
- autism spectrum disorders (including Asperger syndrome)
- behavioural and emotional disorders of children and young people.

A note on learning disability, autism spectrum disorders and dependence on drugs

For the purposes of the MHA and to avoid unnecessary detention, a person with a learning disability (defined as a state of arrested or incomplete development of the mind that includes significant impairment of intelligence and social functioning) must have either:

- abnormally aggressive behaviour, or
- seriously irresponsible conduct

to be detained under the Act. Although these terms are not precisely defined, a number of pointers are given in the Code of Practice to assist practitioners in deciding whether or not these features are present (Department of Health, 2015: Chapter 20).

It should be noted, however, that this so-called 'learning disability qualification' applies only to specific sections of the Act. In particular, it does not apply to detention for assessment under section 2 or detention for less than 72 hours under various other sections (Richards & Moghul, 2010: p. 162).

However the Act's definition of mental disorder does include autism spectrum disorders, including when this occurs together with a learning disability. According to the Code (para. 20.19):

> 'It is possible for someone on the autistic spectrum to meet the criteria in the Act for detention without having any other form of mental disorder, even if the autism is not associated with abnormally aggressive or seriously irresponsible behaviour, but this will be very rare.'

Dependence on alcohol or drugs does not come within the meaning of mental disorder for the purposes of the Act. However, mental disorders that accompany or are associated with the use of or stopping the use of alcohol or drugs, even if they arise from dependence on those substances, may come within the meaning of mental disorder (paras 2.9–2.13).

Criteria for making an application for detention in hospital

Of course, it is not just the definition of mental disorder that is important in deciding whether a person can be detained under the MHA. Certain other criteria must also be met. In brief, the criteria for detention under sections 2 and 3 are that:

▶ the disorder needs to be of a certain nature or degree

▶ the person needs to be in hospital

▶ there is some kind of risk

▶ and, for a section 3, appropriate medical treatment is available.

These criteria are given in full in Box 6.2 and are discussed in more detail later in this chapter.

Process

Section 12 approval

Since April 2013, the Secretary of State, via regional approval panels, has been responsible for the section 12 approval process (prior to this it fell to strategic health authorities). Section 12 of the Act requires that one of the doctors assessing the patient should have special experience in diagnosing and treating mental disorder. Details on how to become a section 12

Box 6.2 Criteria governing applications for detention under the Mental Health Act sections 2 and 3

14.4 A person can be detained for assessment under section 2 only if both the following criteria apply:

- the person is suffering from a mental disorder of a nature or degree which warrants their detention in hospital for assessment (or for assessment followed by treatment) for at least a limited period, and
- the person ought to be so detained in the interests of their own health or safety or with a view to the protection of others.

14.5 A person can be detained for treatment under section 3 only if all the following criteria apply:

- the person is suffering from a mental disorder of a nature or degree which makes it appropriate for them to receive medical treatment in hospital
- it is necessary for the health or safety of the person or for the protection of other persons that they should receive such treatment and it cannot be provided unless the patient is detained under this section, and
- appropriate medical treatment is available.

[Author's note: 'nature' refers to the type of disorder, and 'degree' refers to its severity]

(Department of Health, 2015: p. 113)

approved doctor can be found in Zigmond & Brindle (2016: Chapter 11) and will not be repeated here.

Assessment

▶ In practice, the assessment of a patient under the MHA often begins with a concern raised by a general practitioner, social worker, relative or psychiatrist.

▶ The patient needs to be examined by two doctors (at least one of whom must be section 12 approved) if detention under section 2 or 3 is being considered (the most common situation).

▶ If neither of the doctors has any previous knowledge of the patient, they must both be section 12 approved.

▶ The application is coordinated by the approved mental health professional (AMHP). The doctors must sign their recommendations on or before the AMHP makes the application. The AMHP's application must be made within 14 days of the second medical recommendation.

▶ The assessment interview should be carried out jointly by the AMHP and the two doctors. If this is not possible, both doctors should discuss the patient's case with the AMHP.

▶ The medical recommendations must be made no more than 5 days apart, i.e. there must not be more than 5 clear days between them. They can be made jointly (but beware that any error in a joint recommendation cannot be amended after submission).

▶ The AMHP has powers of conveyance and it is their responsibility to convey the patient to hospital.

▶ The AMHP also has other responsibilities, such as liaising with relatives (although this might also be good practice for the doctors too).

▶ It is the doctors' responsibility to find a bed, and give some thought to the type of bed needed (low secure, intensive care, etc.). NHS England has now made this process national and a single referral form needs to be completed. Although there is a centralised database of the location of beds throughout England, procedures to find a bed when one is needed are still cumbersome and lengthy.

People

The approved clinician (AC)

This term was introduced in 2008, at the same time as the responsible clinician (see below). Approved clinicians can be doctors, psychologists, nurses, occupational therapists or social workers who have been approved on the basis of demonstrated competence in a number of areas described by the Department of Health (2016). Essentially, they involve taking responsibility for the treatment without consent of detained patients, and the list of criteria to fulfil as part of the training requirements is extensive.

Approved clinicians can:

▶ use a section 5(2)

▶ visit and examine patients (section 24)

▶ provide evidence to courts for the forensic sections

▶ provide certificates to authorise treatments under Part IV of the Act

(Richards & Moghul, 2010: p. 128).

The approved clinician need not to be the responsible clinician, although in many cases will be (South London and Maudsley Foundation Trust, 2013: p. 49).

A doctor who becomes approved in this context will automatically also be section 12 approved.

The responsible clinician (RC)

This term replaces responsible medical officer (RMO). A professional, who need not be a doctor, must be an approved clinician before becoming a responsible clinician. All patients detained under the civil or forensic sections of the MHA must have a responsible clinician (except for detentions of brief duration such as for a 5(2), a 5(4) or a 136, each of which is described later in this chapter).

The functions of the responsible clinician include:

▶ having overall responsibility for the care of the patient, including reviewing whether they still need to be detained

▶ granting leave of absence

▶ terminating a section

▶ preventing discharge by a patient's nearest relative

▶ renewing a section and, along with an AMHP, making and recalling patients from community treatment orders (CTOs)

Richards & Moghul (2010: pp. 128–129).

That this role no longer needs to be occupied by a doctor could prove challenging to current custom and practice.

It is possible for a detained patient to have both a responsible clinician and an approved clinician, the latter in charge of one or more aspects of their treatment. This would need to occur, for example, if the responsible clinician was not a doctor and medication was needed.

The approved mental health professional (AMHP)

Since the 2007 amendments to the MHA, professionals other than social workers can enact the functions previously undertaken only by approved social workers (ASW). However, there have been concerns anecdotally about whether there are sufficient numbers of AMHPs available. There was a duty on local authorities to ensure sufficient numbers of ASWs (Care Quality Commission, 2014), but the workforce planning of AMHPs was stipulated in a document published by the National Institute for Mental

Health in England (NIMHE; 2008). The NIMHE is no longer operating, and it is now the responsibility of the local Social Services authority (LSSA) to provide the AMHP service.

The NIMHE guidance (which is still in force) gives detailed information on the role of AMHPs. In summary, they are required to:

▶ take overall responsibility for coordinating the process of MHA assessment
▶ judge whether statutory criteria for detention are met
▶ interview patients appropriately,

in order to:

▶ consider making applications under sections 2, 3, 4 and 7 of the MHA
▶ be involved in all aspects of CTOs and act as a second professional when detentions are to be renewed
▶ under certain circumstances, enter and inspect non-NHS hospitals where a mentally disordered person is a patient if there are concerns about care
▶ apply for a warrant to enter and remove a patient from a specified place, such as their home, under section 135, or to assess with a view to detention under sections 4, 2 or 3
▶ interview a patient who has been removed to a place of safety under sections 135 or 136

(South London and Maudsley Foundation Trust, 2013: p. 44–50).

Note that an AMHP will not make an application for a detention unless an appropriate bed is available for the patient.

Doctors

Otherwise known as the registered medical practitioner (RMP), the role of the doctor clearly has the potential to change in the light of the introduction of the approved clinician and the responsible clinician. However, the medical recommendation for several sections of the MHA needs to be completed by a doctor (see below), and the second opinion appointed doctor (SOAD) is usually an experienced psychiatrist appointed by the CQC to provide a second opinion for the medical treatment of a detained patient (Zigmund & Brindle, 2016: p. 38). Note that there is no legal requirement for any professional involved in the assessment of a young person to be a CAMHS specialist, but the Code of Practice recommends that at least one of the professionals (i.e. one of the two doctors or the AMHP) should have expertise in CAMHS where possible (Barber et al, 2012: p. 135; Department of Health, 2015: para 19.73).

The issue of nominated deputies for section 5(2) is covered in paragraphs 18.12–18.18 of the Code (Department of Health, 2015). It is possible for a registered medical practitioner to choose an approved clinician to be the nominated deputy, but more often the nominated deputy function will fall to the registered medical practitioner on call, that is, a junior doctor. Note that the junior doctor must be registered, i.e. not in their first foundation year. The nominated deputy needs to be on the same staff as the person in charge of the patient's treatment.

In relation to the use of section 5(2) by nominated deputies:

'Doctors and approved clinicians may leave instructions with ward staff to contact them (or their nominated deputy) if a particular patient wants or tries to leave. But they may not leave instructions for their nominated deputy to use section 5, nor may they complete a section 5 report in advance to be used in their absence. The deputy must exercise their own professional judgment' (Department of Health, 2015: para. 18.18).

Hospital managers

Hospital managers have a number of roles in respect of the MHA, including:

- ▶ ensuring the smooth admission and transfer of detained patients
- ▶ the referral of detained patients to mental health tribunals
- ▶ hearing appeals against detention.

Most of their roles are delegated to MHA administrators and nursing staff (Zigmond & Brindle, 2016: pp. 37–38).

Since April 2010, hospital managers have had a new duty to ensure the adequacy of the environment (the so-called age-appropriate environment) for a child or young person admitted formally or informally for a mental disorder under section 131A. The Code of Practice specifies the need for:

- ▶ appropriate physical facilities
- ▶ staff with the appropriate training
- ▶ a hospital routine allowing personal, social and educational development
- ▶ equal access to educational opportunities as peers

(Department of Health, 2015: para. 19.91).

Nearest relative

This is a particular term defined within the MHA, and Chapter 5 of the Code of Practice (Department of Health, 2015) is dedicated to this role. The nearest relative is determined according to a hierarchical list (see below) and is not necessarily the person with parental responsibility (as defined in the Children Act 1989) and vice versa. Unless the patient's parent, spouse or civil partner, the nearest relative must be over 18 years old. If the young person is looked after under a care order or interim care order, then the local authority fulfils this function, and if a child arrangements order is in place, then the nearest relative will be the person named in the order.

The roles and responsibilities of the nearest relative do not apply to restricted patients (those under sections 35, 36 or 38).

The nearest relative:

- can request an assessment to be undertaken for detention in hospital under sections 2, 3 and 4, and in this case becomes 'the applicant' (MHA section 13(4))
- should be informed if a section 2 or section 4 is applied for
- should be consulted before a section 3 or 7 is applied for
- can block the application for a section 3 or 7
- can order the patient's discharge from a section 2 or 3 or a CTO
- should be informed with at least 7 days' notice of a patient's intended discharge or transfer, as long as the patient agrees
- has a right to be invited to a mental health tribunal or hospital managers' hearing.

There is a hierarchical list of who is the nearest relative:

- husband or wife or civil partner
- son or daughter
- father or mother
- brother or sister
- grandparent
- uncle or aunt
- nephew or niece.

The associated rules include that:

- anyone can move to the top of the list if they ordinarily live with or care for the patient; the older person has priority over younger ones
- 'whole-blood' relatives take priority over 'half-blood' ones (if there is more than one person in the category)
- the relative should be ordinarily resident in the UK
- the mother trumps the father if the patient is illegitimate (unless the father has properly established parental responsibility under the Children Act)
- someone who has lived with the patient for at least 5 years can become the nearest relative
- where no obvious nearest relative exists, the county court can appoint one
- the court can also displace the nearest relative if they are thought to be unsuitable, incapable, unreasonably objecting or wish to discharge the patient inappropriately; this procedure can be initiated by the patient, the AMHP or another relative
- the nearest relative can authorise someone else to take on the role, and the designated nearest relative may change if their personal circumstances change

(Harbour, 2008: pp. 64–67; South London and Maudsley Foundation Trust, 2013: pp. 51–58).

It will be noted when comparing the use of sections 2 and 3 that the nearest relative can prevent the application of a section 3, whereas although they might object to a section 2 there are no grounds for them to prevent a section 2 application. This dilemma is discussed by Zigmond & Brindle (2016: pp. 50–51). Although it is not lawful to use a section 2 merely to get around the objections of the nearest relative, and this has been established by case law (South London and Maudsley Foundation Trust, 2013: p. 54), there is an argument that if the nearest relative does object to a section 3, it may not be safe to delay admission while an application to displace the nearest relative is made to the county court (using a section 29).

The request of the nearest relative to discharge a patient is usually made by letter to the hospital. The responsible clinician has 72 hours to decide how to respond. The responsible clinician can prevent the discharge (using a barring order, which can last for 6 months) by completing a form, and the patient and relative should be informed of this. It is possible then for an appeal to be made to a mental health tribunal within 28 days (Richards & Moghul, 2010: p. 125).

If the responsible clinician is considering a barring order, a risk assessment should be performed. The grounds for a barring order are that the responsible clinician thinks that the patient is likely to act in a way that is dangerous to the self or others. A dangerous act is one that is likely to cause serious physical injury or lasting psychological harm (South London and Maudsley Foundation Trust, 2013: p. 57; Department of Health, 2015: Chapter 32; Zigmond & Brindle, 2016: p. 53).

Treatments

What is treatment?

As a general rule, i.e. when we are considering patients not subject to the MHA, it is important to bear in mind that treatment for a physical disorder in someone under 16 can be given under common law (or with parental consent) in an emergency when it is necessary and cannot be delayed. For someone aged 16 and above, treatment for physical disorders in an emergency is now governed by the Mental Capacity Act 2005, which has replaced the common law.

The MHA does not regulate medical treatment for physical health disorders except where they are part of, or ancillary to, a mental disorder (see below).

The longer-term sections, such as section 3, require that appropriate medical treatment be available as one of the criteria for detention.

The amendments to the MHA 1983 listed in Part 1, Chapter 1 of the MHA 2007 describe medical treatment as including 'psychological intervention and specialist mental health habilitation, rehabilitation and care' (section

7(2)) 'the purpose of which is to alleviate, or prevent a worsening of, the disorder or one or more of its symptoms or manifestations' (section 7(3)).

What, it may be asked, is habilitation? Presumably deriving from the Latin *habilitare*, meaning to enable, this is not a term in frequent psychiatric use. In the MHA Code of Practice (Department of Health, 2015: para. 23.2) it is defined as equipping someone with skills and abilities they have never had, as distinct from rehabilitation, which is helping them recover skills and abilities they have lost.

The availability of appropriate medical treatment applies to new assessments under the MHA as well as renewals, for example, of section 3 detentions. It is also a requirement for a CTO, and for mental health tribunals when considering whether or not to discharge patients (Barber *et al*, 2012: p. 24).

The 1983 Act had already specifically mentioned, in section 145, that medical treatment includes nursing. From case law, treatment has been understood as including anything from cure to containment. This is helpfully discussed by Barber *et al* (2012: pp. 25–27): treatment could mean almost anything within this broad spectrum. As these authors highlight, issues concerning availability of treatment may be considered significant. It is not clear whether availability refers to matters of time or place and whether treatment is to be found in the private sector rather than in the NHS. The testing of this requirement is likely to prove of great interest to clinicians.

Treatment in general or psychiatric hospital

Although the MHA makes no distinction between treatment in general or psychiatric hospitals, practitioners should be alert to a couple of points about this. The general hospital needs to have a mechanism of recognising the responsible clinician from a neighbouring organisation (such as a nearby psychiatric hospital). It also needs to have hospital managers who can hear appeals and manage the administrative requirements of the Act. Hospitals in England need to be registered with the CQC to be able to receive detained patients (if not, a patient could not be admitted for treatment under a 5(2), for example).

Treatments needing special measures

Part IV of the MHA (sections 56–64) deals with consent to treatment for detained patients on certain longer-term sections such as section 3. Note that patients on other sections, such as sections 4, 5(2), 5(4), 35, 37, 45, 135 or 136, are not covered by this part of the Act: these patients have the same right to consent to or refuse treatment as anyone not detained under the Act. For the sake of brevity, only sections 57, 58A and 63 will be considered here.

Section 57 treatments refer to the unusual treatment of neurosurgery in which brain tissue is destroyed for the treatment of mental disorder. It also applies to the implantation of sex hormones to reduce male sex drive (Department of Health, 2015: Chapter 24). These treatments need consent and a statutory second opinion (i.e. a panel of three people: a SOAD, plus two non-medical participants). This is required for informal as well as detained patients.

Section 58 deals with medication for mental disorder given more than 3 months after it was first given under detention (the so-called 3-month rule). At this point, either valid consent is needed (as recorded by the responsible clinician or a SOAD) or, if consent cannot be given, the SOAD needs to consult with others and certify that the treatment is appropriate (Department of Health, 2015: Chapter 24).

Treatment using ECT in children and young people is now covered by new safeguards in the 2007 amendments, **section 58A**. These apply regardless of whether or not the young person is detained. A SOAD needs to certify that valid consent has been obtained and that the treatment is appropriate.

Treatment for medical conditions associated with mental disorder

Section 63 allows treatment for mental disorder of detained patients on long-term sections with or without consent. The most common uses of section 63 are for nursing care and to authorise medication in the first 3 months of detention (T. Zigmond, personal communication, 2015). The treatment must be given by or under the direction of the approved clinician in charge of it. There are exclusions to the use of section 63 (neurosurgery, the implantation of hormones and ECT, as described above).

Treatments can be given under section 63 for physical conditions, but only if caused by or a consequence of the mental disorder. The treatment for anorexia nervosa falls within this category, as does the treatment of an overdose of paracetamol or treatment of self-harm. It also covers any investigations needed as part of the treatment of the mental disorder, such as blood tests for lithium or clozapine treatment (Zigmond & Brindle, 2016: p. 78).

The MHA Code of Practice (Department of Health, 2015) emphasises that capacity should still be assessed and consent sought for treatments under this section, even if it isn't legally required.

See Curtice & James (2016) for a brief psychiatric review of the use of section 63 and the range of acts ancillary to the treatment of the mental disorder that have been thought appropriate by the courts and sanctioned.

Some legal experts have voiced concerns about this section and whether it is compatible with ECHR rights and patient autonomy (Jackson, 2013: pp. 324, 355).

The MHA sections in practice

It is helpful to organise this part of the chapter according to the Parts of the MHA (Table 6.1).

Table 6.1 Parts and sections of the Mental Health Act

Part (of 1983 Act as amended in 2007)	Section	Notes
Part I: Application of Act	1	Application of the Act and definitions of mental disorder
Part II: Compulsory admission to hospital and guardianship	2	Admission for assessment
	3	Admission for treatment
	4	Emergency admission for assessment
	5	Application for patient already in hospital
	7	Application for guardianship
	17	Leave of absence
	17A	Community treatment order
Part III: Patients concerned in criminal proceedings or under sentence	35–55	Patients involved in criminal justice system
Part IV: Consent to treatment	56–64	Consent to treatment
Part V: Mental health review tribunals (now renamed in England)	65–79	Mental health tribunals
Part VIII: Miscellaneous functions	117	Aftercare
Part X: Miscellaneous and supplementary	131	Informal admission of patients
	131A	The duty of managers to ensure an age-appropriate environment
	135	Warrant to search for and remove patients
	136	Mentally disordered persons found in public places

▶ Part I, section 1 deals with definitions of the Act and these have been dealt with above.

▶ Part II, sections 2, 3, 4, 5(2), 5(4), 7, 17 and 17A are described below.

▶ Part III concerns the forensic sections, which are covered in Chapter 8.

▶ Part IV is about consent: see Chapter 4 and above.

▶ Part V is about mental health tribunals. As these are covered in other texts (e.g. Zigmond & Brindle, 2016) and the same rules apply as for adults, they will not be dealt with here. One change from 2007 must be mentioned: children and young people subject to the MHA must now be referred to a tribunal hearing after 1 year (as opposed to after 3 years for adults).

▶ Part VIII, section 117 concerns aftercare and is briefly mentioned below.

▶ Part X, section 131, concerning admission, is described below; section 131A is the duty of managers to ensure appropriate environments, as described above (p. 74); sections 135 and 136 are also described below.

Part II sections

Section 2: Admission for assessment

For what? The detention and treatment in hospital for up to 28 days of a patient believed to have a mental disorder.

For whom? A patient who fulfils the criteria for an application under section 2, namely:

▶ the person is suffering from a mental disorder of a nature or degree that warrants their detention in hospital for assessment (or for assessment followed by treatment) for at least a limited period, and

▶ the person ought to be so detained in the interests of their own health or safety, or to protect others.

Nature refers to the type of disorder, and degree refers to its severity.

What can be done? Detention; if the person absconds, forced return by any staff member or by the police; treatment for mental disorder with or without their consent.

Who is needed? Two doctors and an AMHP (or, unusually, the nearest relative). One of the doctors must be section 12 approved. One doctor should know the patient, if possible. The recommendations can be made separately or jointly, but each person must interview the patient, and one must discuss the patient with the applicant. (Note that errors on joint applications cannot be corrected after submission, but errors on single ones can be.) There must be no more than 5 days between the medical recommendations.

For how long? For up to 28 days. The person must be admitted to hospital within 14 days of the last-dated medical interview. A section 2 cannot be renewed, but could be replaced by a section 3 if necessary. It can be terminated by the responsible clinician before the end of the 28 days; or the patient can be discharged by a mental health tribunal, by a hospital managers' hearing or by the nearest relative. As with other sections, it is not considered good practice to allow it to lapse.

Anything else? There are rights of appeal. Patients can request the presence of another person, such as an advocate, at the assessment. The application can be made by either an AMHP or the nearest relative.

Unlike a section 3, the nearest relative cannot object to a section 2.

There should be no conflicts of interest among the doctors and AMHP, for example they should not be related, have any business interests skewing their judgement or one should not be line managed by the other.

Patients can be transferred between hospitals using a section 19 (this is a section for just this purpose: doctors do not have to be involved with it).

Leave can be allowed by the responsible clinician, who completes a section 17 form.

Rectifiable errors include misspelled names, or errors in places or dates. It is not permissible to fail to sign the form, or to have a medical recommendation dated after the application date. Problems can occur if a bed is not available at the time of the assessment: in this case, the AMHP will be unwilling to complete their part of the application, and a reassessment by the AMHP will be needed as soon as a bed can be found.

Section 3: Admission for treatment

For what? The detention and treatment of a patient in hospital for up to 6 months.

For whom? A patient who fulfils the criteria for an application under section 3, namely:

- ▶ the person is suffering from a mental disorder of a nature or degree that warrants their detention in hospital for treatment, and
- ▶ it is necessary for the health or safety of the person or for the protection of others that they receive medical treatment, appropriate treatment is available and it cannot be provided unless the person is detained under this section.

What can be done? Detention; if the person absconds, forced return by any staff member or by the police; treatment for mental disorder with or without their consent.

Who is needed? Two doctors and an AMHP (or, unusually, the nearest relative). One of the doctors must be section 12 approved. One doctor should know the patient, if possible. The recommendations can be made separately or jointly, but each person must interview the patient, and one must discuss the patient with the applicant. (Note that errors on joint applications cannot be corrected after submission, but errors on single ones can be.) There must be no more than 5 days between the medical recommendations.

For how long? For up to 6 months. The person must be admitted to hospital within 14 days of the last-dated medical interview.

The section can be renewed for a further 6-month period. Subsequent renewals are possible for up to 1 year at a time, but need another professional's opinion as well as personal examination by the responsible clinician: renewal criteria are the same as the criteria for initial detention.

The section can be terminated by the responsible clinician before the end of the 6 months; or the patient can be discharged by a mental health tribunal, by a hospital managers' hearing or by the nearest relative. It can also be transferred into a community treatment order (CTO). As with other sections, it is not considered good practice to allow it to lapse.

Anything else? There are rights of appeal. Patients can request the presence of another person, such as an advocate, at the assessment. The application can be made by either an AMHP or the nearest relative.

The nearest relative can object to a section 3 application.

There should be no conflicts of interest among the doctors and AMHP, for example they should not be related, have any business interests skewing their judgement or one should not be line managed by the other.

Patients can be transferred between hospitals using section 19.

Leave can be allowed by the responsible clinician, who completes a section 17 form.

Rectifiable errors include misspelled names, or errors in places or dates. It is not permissible to fail to sign the form, or to have a medical recommendation dated after the application date.

Section 4: Emergency admission for assessment

For what? The admission and detention of a patient in hospital for up to 72 hours when two doctors are not available for a section 2 application and urgent admission is needed.

For whom? A patient who fulfils the criteria for an application under section 2, namely:

▶ the person is suffering from a mental disorder of a nature or degree that warrants their detention in hospital for assessment (or for assessment followed by treatment) for at least a limited period, and

▶ the person ought to be so detained in the interests of their own health or safety, or to protect others, and

▶ compliance with requirements for section 2 would involve undesirable delay.

What can be done? Admission and detention; if the person absconds, forced return by any staff member or by the police; if the young person is over 16 and lacks capacity, the Mental Capacity Act can be used; if under 16, parental consent or common law can be used.

Who is needed? One doctor and an AMHP (or, unusually, the nearest relative). The doctor should know the patient if possible, but does not need to be section 12 approved or an approved clinician. The recommendation needs to state that an emergency exists, that a (specified) delay would otherwise be caused, and that the delay might result in harm to the patient or to others.

For how long? For up to 72 hours. The AMHP should have seen the patient during the previous 24 hours. The person must be admitted to hospital within 24 hours of the earliest of either recommendation and the 72 hours begins on admission.

The section cannot be renewed, but could be replaced by a section 2 with a second medical recommendation. In this case, the duration of the section 2 begins from the start of the section 4. However, if a section 3 is being considered, two new medical recommendations are needed.

The section is terminated either when assessment finds that the criteria for a 2 or a 3 are not met, or when the 72 hours end. As with other sections, it is not considered good practice to allow it to lapse.

Anything else? There are rights of appeal, but owing to the temporary nature of this section the mental health tribunal will normally await further developments (conversion to a section 2 or 3) before acting.

No leave applies.

Section 5(2): Application by a doctor for a patient already in hospital

For what? The detention of a voluntary patient in hospital by any doctor or approved clinician for up to 72 hours.

For whom? A voluntary in-patient (i.e. a patient in hospital already, not an out-patient or anyone attending an emergency department) who it seems likely would be eligible for an application under a section 2 or 3.

What can be done? Detention; if the person absconds, forced return by any staff member or by the police. Treatment cannot be authorised with this section: if the young person is over 16 and lacks capacity, the MCA can be used; if under 16, parental consent or common law can be used.

Who is needed? A doctor or approved clinician in charge of the patient's treatment or the nominated deputy of either (for nominated deputies see p. 73).

For how long? For up to 72 hours to allow sufficient time for an application for a longer section if needed. A section 5(2) cannot be renewed. It ends when it is decided that an assessment for a section 2 or 3 is not required; or it lapses (which is not considered good practice) or the patient is moved from the hospital.

Anything else? The patient should have been examined by the doctor or approved clinician and a report stating that informal treatment is no longer appropriate needs to be handed to the hospital managers. The doctor can be the ward doctor.

It is not lawful for a note to be left stating 'if the patient leaves put on a section 5(2)', as case law has established that this sways the judgement of staff (*R (ZN) v South West London & St George's Mental Health NHS Trust* (2009)).

Patients cannot be transferred to another hospital under this section (Department of Health, 2015: paras 18.42–18.45).

No leave is allowed.

The MHA Code of Practice (Department of Health, 2015: para 18.11) states that a doctor using this power on a patient not under the care of a psychiatrist should seek the advice of a psychiatrist (or approved clinician) to obtain confirmation of their opinion that the patient does need to be so detained.

Section 5(4): Application by a nurse for a patient already in hospital

For what? The emergency detention of a voluntary patient in hospital by a nurse for up to 6 hours when a section 5(2) application cannot be made in time.

For whom? A voluntary in-patient (i.e. a patient in hospital already) receiving treatment for a mental disorder, when it appears that the disorder is such that it is necessary for the patient's health or safety or the protection of others that they are restrained from leaving hospital.

What can be done? Detention; if the person absconds, forced return by any staff member or by the police; treatment cannot be authorised with this section unless the person can consent to it.

Who is needed? A registered mental health or learning disabilities nurse.

For how long? For up to 6 hours. This cannot be renewed. It ends either when a section 5(2) is applied instead (in which case the 6 hours of the section 5(4) is included in the 72 hours of the 5(2)) or it when lapses (which is not considered good practice).

Anything else? Patients cannot be transferred to another hospital under this section. If they are, the section ceases.

Section 7: Application for guardianship

As this is understood to be in decline, and as it is available only for young people over the age of 16, it will not be dealt with here.

Other sections

Section 17: Leave of absence

Section 17 leave can only be granted by the responsible clinician, or in their absence (e.g. if they are on leave) by the approved clinician who is standing in for them (Department of Health, 2015: para. 27.8). It is important to know that this responsibility cannot otherwise be delegated. In particular, it is unlawful to write 'leave at nurses' discretion' on the file, but it is possible to specify in advance that leave can be withdrawn at the nurses' discretion.

Trainees cannot grant section 17 leave.

The MHA requires that a CTO should be considered for leave longer than 7 days.

Section 17 leave is needed if a patient is to attend a general hospital for treatment of a physical disorder, or to attend sites managed by a different NHS trust.

Note that if it is to be granted to patients on certain forensic sections (see Chapter 8), the approval of the Secretary of State is needed.

Section 17A: Community treatment orders

For what? The community-based treatment of a patient who has already been detained (on a section 3 for example). The community treatment order can be made for up to 6 months, and can then be renewed for a further period of up to 6 months and then annually.

For whom? For patients who have already been detained on certain sections (3, 37, 45A, 47 or 48) and:

▶ the person is suffering from a mental disorder of a nature or degree that makes it appropriate for them to receive medical treatment, and

▶ it is necessary for the health or safety of the person or for the protection of others that they should receive such treatment, and

▶ such treatment can be provided without detaining the person in hospital, and

▶ the responsible clinician can exercise the power of recall to hospital, and

▶ appropriate medical treatment is available.

What can be done? Recall to hospital. The consent to treatment provisions are complex and covered in Chapter 8 of Zigmond & Brindle (2016).

There are two mandatory conditions:

▶ the patient must make themselves available for examination by the responsible clinician, and

▶ the patient must make themselves available for examination by the SOAD.

In addition, various discretionary conditions can be applied with the aim of ensuring that the patient receives treatment, of preventing harm and protecting others (but not amounting to a deprivation of liberty).

Who is needed? The responsible clinician and an AMHP.

For how long? There is no time limit imposed on when the forms should be completed by the responsible clinician and the AMHP. The order ends by discharge by the responsible clinician; by recall and revocation; or by discharge by a mental health tribunal, a hospital managers' hearing or the nearest relative. As with other sections, it is not considered good practice to allow it to lapse. Within the final 2 months, a decision can be made about renewal for a further 6 months and, thereafter, yearly.

Anything else? There are rights of appeal. No leave applies. The recall procedure can be enacted by the responsible clinician if:

► the patient requires medical treatment in hospital for mental disorder and

► there would be a risk of harm to the health or safety of the patient or to others if the patient were not recalled for treatment

or

► the patient fails to comply with either of the mandatory conditions.

If the patient happens to be in hospital as an in-patient when recalled, a 5(2) cannot be used. There is a procedure for recall that includes delivery of a specific form to the patient's address. A 72-hour period begins on arrival in hospital to assess whether the CTO should be revoked (in which case the previous section is reactivated from the start) or the patient released.

Section 117: Aftercare

All patients who have been detained under section 3, 37, 45, 47 or 48 are entitled to aftercare free of charge. The MHA Code of Practice (Department of Health, 2015) recommends that aftercare should be broadly defined. From paragraph 33.4 of the Code, it might include:

> 'healthcare, social care and employment services, supported accommodation and services to meet the person's wider social, cultural and spiritual needs, if these services meet a need that arises directly from or is related to the particular patient's mental disorder, and help to reduce the risk of deterioration in the patient's mental condition.'

Aftercare should continue for as long as the patient needs it.

Section 131: Informal admission of patients

Section 131 is an interesting inclusion in the Act, and one wonders why it is there at all. It is very likely to lead to understandable confusion. This is demonstrated in one text (Maden & Spencer-Lane, 2010: p. 127), which stipulates that 'If admission is informal, age 16+, use section 131 of the Mental Health Act'. As if that was all that was needed. The following is the verbatim section of the Act (the square brackets indicate the 2007 amendments):

> '131 **Informal admission of patients.**
>
> (1) Nothing in this Act shall be construed as preventing a patient who requires treatment for mental disorder from being admitted to any hospital or [F1registered establishment] in pursuance of arrangements made in that behalf and without any application, order or direction rendering him liable to be detained under this Act, or from remaining in any hospital or [F1registered establishment] in pursuance of such arrangements after he has ceased to be so liable to be detained.

[F2(2)Subsections (3) and (4) below apply in the case of a patient aged 16 or 17 years who has capacity to consent to the making of such arrangements as are mentioned in subsection (1) above.

(3) If the patient consents to the making of the arrangements, they may be made, carried out and determined on the basis of that consent even though there are one or more persons who have parental responsibility for him.

(4) If the patient does not consent to the making of the arrangements, they may not be made, carried out or determined on the basis of the consent of a person who has parental responsibility for him.

(5) In this section—

(a) the reference to a patient who has capacity is to be read in accordance with the Mental Capacity Act 2005; and

(b) "parental responsibility" has the same meaning as in the Children Act 1989.]'

Section 131 (subsections 3–5) apply only to young people above 16 years of age. The section covers admission: it is not intended to cover treatment for either physical disorders or mental disorder. And it only applies to young people who have capacity as defined in the MCA (see Chapter 7).

So in an Act that, in the mind of clinicians, is all about detention and compulsory treatment, why is there a section about informal admission? Historically, this section appears to be a vestige from the Percy Commission review in the 1950s (for a synopsis of the statutory history of this section as discussed during the Bournewood case, see Kennedy & Grubb, 2000: p. 906). The Percy Commission was concerned at that time with the large number of patients detained in mental deficiency hospitals: it recommended that compulsory powers should be used only when absolutely necessary. Allowing patients with mental illness or mental deficiency to be in hospital without using compulsory powers was seen as desirable.

Prior to the 2007 amendments, section 131(2) allowed for the admission of young people who could express their own wishes and consent to admission, irrespective of the wishes of those with parental responsibility. The effect of the amendments is to change the emphasis, and this is why it is of interest to us here. The change means that young people of 16 and 17 with a mental disorder can only be admitted to hospital if they have capacity and can consent, but they specifically cannot be so admitted on the basis of parental consent alone.

For matters relating to consent concerning admission to hospital for treatment, see Chapter 4.

Section 135(1): Warrant to search for and remove patients

For what? The power to enter private property to remove a patient to a place of safety (usually hospital) for assessment for up to 72 hours.

For whom? A patient who appears to a magistrate to:

▶ be suffering from a mental disorder

- have been or be being ill-treated, neglected or kept otherwise than under proper control, or
- be living alone and unable to care for themselves.

What can be done? Entry to look for the person (once only); removal of the person to a place of safety; detention; if the person absconds, forced return by any staff member or by the police; treatment cannot be authorised with this section unless the person can consent to it.

Who is needed? An AMHP applies to a magistrate, who issues a section 135(1) warrant, and a police officer is thereby authorised to enter locked premises if necessary to remove the person.

The police officer must be accompanied by an AMHP and a doctor (who should be section 12 approved or an approved clinician).

For how long? For up to 72 hours from the time of admission to the place of safety. The warrant must be used within 1 month. Section 135 cannot be renewed, but could be replaced by a section 2 or 3 before its expiry. The section is terminated either when assessment finds that the criteria for a section 2 or 3 are not met, or the 72 hours end. As with other sections, it is not considered good practice to allow it to lapse.

Anything else? There are no rights of appeal and no leave applies. Patients can be transferred between places of safety.

Section 135(2) concerns the authorising of a police officer by a magistrate to find someone already detained under the MHA.

Section 136: Mentally disordered persons found in public places

Some background

At the time of writing, the detention of children and young people on a section 136 in police cells has been very topical. The Association of Chief Police Officers estimated that 580 individuals under the age of 18 were detained under section 136 in 2012–2013; of those, it was estimated that 263 (45%) were taken into police custody (Health Select Committee, 2014). This matter has provoked much debate, with the Royal College of Psychiatrists as well as Members of Parliament calling for a swift end to the practice.

This use of section 136 was in fact highlighted by the House of Commons Health Select Committee in its report on the legislative amendments introduced by the MHA 2007:

> 'The Committee recommends that the Department of Health reviews as a matter of urgency the practice of detaining children under section 136 and, that as part of the review, it examines the outcomes for children detained in this way. This review should be undertaken with a view to identifying effective alternative options that can be used by the police and health care professionals' (Health Select Committee, 2013: para. 15, p. 40).

The Committee's findings were included in a review of the operation of sections 135 and 136 published by the Department of Health & Home Office (2014). Recommendations include amending the legislation so that children and young people aged under 18 are never taken to police cells if detained under section 135 or 136; reducing the maximum length of detention from 72 to 24 hours; operating street triage (where the police on the scene can call on the advice of a mental health nurse); and widening the concept of places of safety to include community settings.

The MHA Code of Practice for England (Department of Health, 2015) is quite clear on the use of police stations in the case of section 136 (but note that there are some slight differences in the Code of Practice for Wales (Welsh Assembly Government, 2008)). It stipulates that police cells should be used only in exceptional circumstances when the behaviour of an individual appearing to suffer from a mental disorder poses an unmanageably high risk to others (para. 16.38). Indeed, the whole of Chapter 16 of the Code is about the use of this particular police power, perhaps reflecting public concern about its implementation.

Two publications from the Royal College of Psychiatrists are relevant to places of safety: a college report from 2011 and a position statement from 2013. The college report (Royal College of Psychiatrists, 2011) outlines standards and makes recommendations on staffing levels and competencies required of the staff involved. The position statement (Royal College of Psychiatrists, 2013: p. 4) stipulates the following:

'1 The custody suite should be used in exceptional circumstances only.

2 A vehicle supplied by the ambulance provider should be able to attend promptly so that it is used for conveyance unless the person is too disturbed.

3 The AMHP and doctor approved under Section 12(2) of the Mental Health Act should attend within 3 h in all cases where there are not good clinical grounds to delay assessment.

4 The first doctor to perform a Mental Health Act assessment should be approved under Section 12(2) of the Act.

5 A monitoring form should be agreed locally to meet all the national requirements and should be completed in all cases.

6 Commissioners should ensure that there is a multi-agency group meeting to develop, implement and quality assure the agreed policy. This group should review the monitoring data. It should also consider how the need for use of Section 136 might be reduced.'

Although discussion of the clinical characteristics of adolescents placed on a section 136 is beyond the scope of this book, a survey by Patil *et al* (2013) of 40 adolescents detained in London between 2007 and 2010 (excluding those detained in police cells) revealed a vulnerable group with high rates of abuse and institutionalisation. Only half were subsequently admitted to hospital. However, this low admission rate might reflect a scarcity of facilities. The College's Faculty of Child and Adolescent Psychiatry has also developed a draft position statement on distinguishing a health-based place of safety, for the purposes of section 136 assessment, from a crisis assessment site (Fellow-Smith *et al*, 2016). This is in response to an increased focus on the need to clarify crisis care in England and Wales.

Let us now look at the basics of section 136.

For what? The power for a police officer to remove a patient who appears to be suffering from a mental disorder from a public place to a place of safety (usually hospital) for assessment for up to 72 hours.

For whom? A patient who appears to a police officer to:

▶ be suffering from a mental disorder, and
▶ to be in immediate need of care or control,

such that the police officer considers it necessary in the person's interests or for the protection of others to remove them to a place of safety.

What can be done? Detention; if the person absconds, forced return by any staff member or by the police; treatment cannot be authorised with this section unless the person can consent to it.

Who is needed? A police officer.

For how long? For up to 72 hours from the time of arrival at the place of safety.

A section 136 cannot be renewed. A section 2 or 3 can be initiated before it lapses, if required.

Both a doctor (who should be section 12 approved) and an AMHP are required to assess the patient within 72 hours. If they do not think there are grounds for conversion to a section 2 or 3, the section 136 will terminate.

Anything else? There are no rights of appeal and no leave applies.

Patients can be transferred between places of safety.

The MHA Code of Practice stipulates that the assessment should begin as soon as possible after arrival of the patient and that it is good practice that this is within 3 hours (Department of Health, 2015: para 16.47). If the detention is in a police cell, then it should be for no more than 24 hours (para. 16.40).

It will be of interest and concern to clinicians that in an adult case (*MS v UK* (2012)), a patient with a mental illness was successful in arguing that his ECHR Article 3 rights were violated for the time he spent in a police cell under section 136. He was in the cell for more than 72 hours, during which time he was without treatment. Even though the aunt with whom he lived had sustained severe injuries during the assault that led to the patient's removal to the police station, he was not charged. Apparently, psychiatrists were assuming that he would be charged and the search for a bed was delayed on this account; when charges were not pressed, attempts to find a bed in an intensive or medium secure setting were not successful within the 72-hour period.

This returns us to the matter of bed searching and the introductory paragraphs of this chapter. Section 140 of the MHA specifies that health authorities have a duty to inform Social Services which hospitals provide beds for urgent admissions and also which have facilities suitable for the admission of individuals under the age of 18. The Code of Practice also specifies (in para. 14.89) the need for bed managers to work closely with commissioners.

Conclusion

This chapter has described the changes made to the MHA by the 2007 amendments, with particular emphasis on how these affect children and young people. Figures about how widely the MHA is used for individuals under 18 years of age are hard to find and need to be better available to enable study of the changing use of the Act with this age group. The topics discussed have included the principles of the Act, the process of detention and the key roles of the participants. Treatments are dealt with in brief, and finally practical aspects of the sections of the Act are summarised with particular notes on sections 131 and 136.

It is possible that some changes to the Act will be recommended in the current Law Commission review (Law Commission, 2015). It is also to be hoped that improvements can be made to the system of trying to located tier 4 beds for children and young people who need them closer to their homes.

CHAPTER 7

The Mental Capacity Act

The Mental Capacity Act 2005 (MCA) became law in England and Wales in April 2007. It is an Act applying to anyone over the age of 16 who lacks capacity to make decisions for themselves about matters concerning their welfare, finances or health.

Although the Act is widely seen as 'inclusive and patient-friendly' when compared with the Mental Health Act (Jackson, 2013: p. 289), the sections relating to the Deprivation of Liberty Safeguards (DoLS) and the new Schedules have had a very different reception. These were introduced by an amendment to the Mental Health Act in 2007, and came into effect in 2009. For example one senior judge, Lady Hale, wrote:

> 'It is not just the length of the Schedules which makes them so impenetrable, but their obscure language, their relentless over-specification of detail, and their convoluted structure which makes it impossible to find the answer to any question in any one place' (cited in Jackson, 2013: p. 310).

The MCA created a new Court of Protection in England (there was prior to this a Court of Protection existing as part of the Supreme Court). The Court of Protection makes decisions about the personal welfare and financial affairs of people who lack capacity.

Although the MCA as a whole is held in high regard – according to the House of Lords Select Committee's post-legislative scrutiny report (House of Lords, 2014) – considerable problems have been acknowledged with it. These include much misunderstanding of the Act, little ownership of it and poor implementation. The DoLS in particular attracted so much criticism that the Committee thought the only recommendation they could make was to 'start again'. Jones, in the preface to the sixth edition of his *Mental Capacity Act Manual*, is highly critical and highlights a particular concern that case law developing from the DoLs is rendering the notion of liberty meaningless (Jones, 2014: pp. v–vi).

The difficulty for clinicians in child mental health is that this Act adds a layer of complexity to the other legislation to be considered, namely the Mental Health Act 1983 (as amended in 2007) and the Children Act 1989 (as amended in 2004), without offering clear guidelines about what to do when a young person's treatment might involve a deprivation of liberty.

At first glance, child psychiatrists may wonder how relevant the MCA is for their everyday practice. A brief survey of cases heard in the Court of Protection in England and Wales (as published on BAILII for 2015, for example) reveals that few cases involving young people reach the Court: most were about the affairs and property of older adults lacking capacity. Cases involving young people who lack capacity to make decisions can be heard in the Court of Protection and also in the Family Division of the High Court. Cases can be transferred from one court to the other.

It is relevant to be reminded that:

▶ the DoLS do not apply to young people under 18

▶ no one under 18 can make a valid advance decision to refuse treatment (in the terms of the MCA)

▶ no one under 18 can make, or be appointed under, a lasting power of attorney

▶ no one under 18 can be appointed a deputy, for the purpose of the MCA.

What the MCA is supposed to do is provide a framework for giving care and treatment to individuals who lack capacity as defined in the Act, but who do not fall within the scope of the MHA (see Chapter 6). For elderly people with cognitive impairment receiving care for physical disorders, this is obviously sensible. However, in the case of young people aged 16–18 the situation is less clear.

Is capacity the same as or distinct from competence? Although the terms capacity and competence are used interchangeably by some (e.g. Kennedy & Grubb, 2000: p. 596), capacity is best thought of as a legal concept with application to young people above the age of 16, as defined in the MCA. Competence should be reserved to describe the presence of sufficient understanding and intelligence in a child younger than 16 (as in Gillick competence, discussed in Chapter 4).

Where do the so-called Deprivation of Liberty Safeguards fit into the Act? As mentioned in Chapters 1 and 2, there has been much discussion about the concept of deprivation of liberty in light of the European Convention on Human Rights (ECHR), which forms that basis of the Human Rights Act 1998. The Deprivation of Liberty Safeguards were introduced into the MCA in 2007 (and implemented in April 2009) following a European Court of Human Rights decision about the so-called Bournewood case, known more accurately as *HL v UK* (2004).

This case concerned a man with a learning (intellectual) disability and autism, who lacked capacity to consent to his admission to a psychiatric hospital and treatment. This deprivation of his liberty was found to breach Article 5 of the ECHR: the right to liberty and security of person.

The introduction of a framework for lawfully depriving people of their liberty has been seen as a protection for the vulnerable, but is also fraught with practical problems, and the procedures are slow, expensive and not considered effective (Penny & Exworthy, 2015). It is understood that there are wide variations in applying them in practice. These safeguards were intended for people with dementia, severe learning disability or neurological conditions, not for people who would otherwise be detained under the MHA.

It is fortunate in some ways that, although the MCA applies to everyone over the age of 16, the DoLS do not apply to anyone under the age of 18. They will therefore not be further discussed here. They have, in any case, been widely thought unfit for purpose and in need of reform. What this means, however, is that there is a current gap in the statutory provisions for treating in in-patient units young people between the ages of 16 and 18 who lack capacity and who are not detained under the MHA. This is of some legitimate concern.

While that gap persists, the courts can make welfare orders through the Court of Protection for certain cases. These might include, for example, cases in which treatments are needed that involve a deprivation of liberty, or where there are disagreements over a young person's best interests or capacity. Courts can also make orders using their powers under the inherent jurisdiction. It seems likely that, in the near future, amendments will be made to the statutory provision in an attempt to close this gap (via the protective care scheme – see Chapter 1).

This chapter, then, deals only with selected parts of the MCA as applicable to young people between the ages of 16 and 18. First, I outline the Act itself – its general principles, definitions, decision-making, best interests and Section 5 acts. Next, I discuss the assessment of capacity and how this was derived. Finally, I explore the application of the MCA, also considering the relationship between the MCA and the MHA, highlighting material from the MCA Code of Practice.

A note on the MCA Code of Practice

The Code of Practice for the MCA (Department for Constitutional Affairs, 2007), in the same way as the Code of Practice for the MHA (Department of Health, 2015), is not legally binding, but all professionals must have regard to it and give good reasons to justify why they have not followed it (Department for Constitutional Affairs, 2007: p. 1). It differs from the MHA Code, however, in that it applies to both England and Wales.

Although only applicable to young people between the ages of 16 and 18, an entire chapter of the Code (Chapter 12) is dedicated to them. In the Code, a child is anyone under 16 and a young person is anyone between 16 and 18. Relevant sections of the Code will be examined later in this chapter (pp. 102–104).

Table 7.1 Sections of the Mental Capacity Act directly relevant to young people

Part	Section	Notes
Part I	1	Principles
	2	People who lack capacity
	3	Inability to make decisions
	4	Best interests
	4A, 4B	Restriction on deprivation of liberty and deprivation of liberty necessary for life-sustaining treatment
	5	Acts in connection with care or treatment
	6	Section 5 acts: limitations
	27	Family relationships, etc.
	28	Mental Health Act matters
	44	Ill-treatment or neglect

The MCA and relevant sections

The MCA is divided into three parts: Part 1 concerns persons who lack capacity; Part 2 deals with the functions of the Court of Protection and the office of the Public Guardian; Part 3 covers the 'miscellaneous and general'. Parts 2 and 3 do not concern us here. Table 7.1 outlines the sections with which we will be concerned.

Section 1: Principles

(1) The following principles apply for the purposes of this Act.

(2) A person must be assumed to have capacity unless it is established that he lacks capacity.

(3) A person is not to be treated as unable to make a decision unless all practicable steps to help him to do so have been taken without success.

(4) A person is not to be treated as unable to make a decision merely because he makes an unwise decision.

(5) An act done, or decision made, under this Act for or on behalf of a person who lacks capacity must be done, or made, in his best interests.

(6) Before the act is done, or the decision is made, regard must be had to whether the purpose for which it is needed can be as effectively achieved in a way that is less restrictive of the person's rights and freedom of action.

(Mental Capacity Act 2005: Part 1, sections 1(1)–1(6))

Section 2: People who lack capacity

(1) For the purposes of this Act, a person lacks capacity in relation to a matter if at the material time he is unable to make a decision for himself in relation to the matter because of an impairment of, or a disturbance in the functioning of, the mind or brain.

(2) It does not matter whether the impairment or disturbance is permanent or temporary.

(3) A lack of capacity cannot be established merely by reference to –

   (a) a person's age or appearance, or

   (b) a condition of his, or an aspect of his behaviour, which might lead others to make unjustified assumptions about his capacity.

(4) In proceedings under this Act or any other enactment, any question whether a person lacks capacity within the meaning of this Act must be decided on the balance of probabilities.

(5) No power which a person ("D") may exercise under this Act –

   (a) in relation to a person who lacks capacity, or

   (b) where D reasonably thinks that a person lacks capacity,

is exercisable in relation to a person under 16.

(Mental Capacity Act 2005: Part 1, sections 2(1)–2(5))

Section 3: Inability to make decisions

The MCA defines this negatively and in a rather confusing way. Thus, a person is unable to make decisions for himself if he is unable:

   '(a) to understand the information relevant to the decision,

   (b) to retain that information,

   (c) to use or weigh that information as part of the process of making the decision, or

   (d) to communicate his decision (whether by talking, using sign language or any other means)' (section 3(1)(a)–(d)).

This section continues:

'A person is not to be regarded as unable to understand the information relevant to a decision if he is able to understand an explanation of it given to him in a way that is appropriate to his circumstances (using simple language, visual aids or any other means)' (section 3(2)).

Nor does it matter if he only retains the information for a short time.

Section 4: Best interests

This was a phrase already in existence from common law. Section 4 lists a number of factors that must hold in the making of a best interests decision, including:

- ▶ the absence of assumptions
- ▶ all relevant circumstances must be considered, including whether the person is likely to have capacity at some stage
- ▶ the person must be encouraged to participate
- ▶ the person's past and present wishes, feelings, beliefs and values must be considered
- ▶ the views of anyone named as important to the person (such as a carer) must be considered.

Note that the both the British Medical Association (2010: p. 19 & p. 47) and the General Medical Council (2007: p. 7 & p. 13) provide versions of this best interests checklist for the four nations (England, Wales, Scotland and Northern Ireland). The BMA's list includes clinical judgement and the risks and side-effects of treatment.

Sections 4A (restriction on deprivation of liberty) and 4B (deprivation of liberty necessary for life-sustaining treatment etc.)

These sections were inserted as a result of the European Court of Human Rights' decision in the Bournewood case (see p. 93 above). Both concern the deprivation of liberty. Section 4A allows one person to deprive another of their liberty only when authorised by a court. Section 4B states the conditions that must be met to allow the deprivation of liberty in order to provide life-sustaining treatment. Neither is applicable to individuals under 18.

Section 5: Acts in connection with care or treatment

This concerns liability for acts done under the MCA. Essentially, the Act allows a practitioner to give a person treatment for a physical disorder without consent as long as they believe that the person lacks capacity and their intended treatment is in the person's best interests. Negligent acts are clearly not protected.

Acts that fall into this category are listed in the Code of Practice (Department for Constitutional Affairs, 2007: Chapter 6). These might include help with washing, eating and communication, carrying out diagnostic investigations, and giving dental treatment or medication. Decisions of greater import require a more elaborate documentation process (Brindle *et al*, 2015: p. 21).

Section 6: Limitations on Section 5 acts

This section concerns restraint. The Act stipulates that, in order to be protected from liability in restraining a person who lacks capacity, the healthcare provider (say) must believe that the restraint is necessary to prevent harm to the person and that the restraint used is proportionate to the likelihood and seriousness of harm. The Code of Practice suggests that professionals should also be aware of professional guidance about this

(Department for Constitutional Affairs, 2007: paras 6.41 and 6.42). Note also that section 6 (and Chapter 6 of the Code) stipulates that protection for health professionals does not extend to any act that constitutes a deprivation of liberty.

Section 27: Family relationships etc.

This is a section stipulating that nothing in the Act permits anyone to make a decision on anyone else's behalf about certain key matters:

▶ consent to marriage or civil partnership

▶ consent to sexual relations

▶ consent to a divorce or dissolution order based on 2 years' separation

▶ consent to a child's being placed for adoption or to the making of an adoption order

▶ discharging parental responsibilities in matters not relating to a child's property.

Section 28: Mental Health Act matters

Concerning the treatment of patients who are also detained under the MHA, section 28 of the MCA stipulates that:

'(1) Nothing in this Act authorises anyone–

(a) to give a patient medical treatment for mental disorder, or

(b) to consent to a patient's being given medical treatment for mental disorder,

if, at the time when it is proposed to treat the patient, his treatment is regulated by Part 4 [Part IV] of the Mental Health Act.'

In other words, if a patient is detained under the MHA and Part IV applies (for example, they are on one of the longer-term sections such as a section 3), then the MCA cannot be used to treat them for mental disorder.

The MCA can, however, be used for the treatment of a physical disorder not related to the mental disorder if the person lacks capacity (Puri *et al*, 2012: p. 149). For other matters concerning the relationship between the two Acts, see pp. 104–106 below.

For patients detained on MHA sections 4, 5(2), 5(4), 35, 135(1) and 136 there is no authority to treat using the powers of the MHA. Therefore, treatment of mental or physical disorders could be given to such people using the MCA if they lack capacity and refused it.

Section 44: Ill-treatment or neglect

Section 44 creates a new offence of ill-treatment by a person if they neglect or ill-treat someone who lacks capacity. This does apply to children under 16. The Code of Practice (Department for Constitutional Affairs, 2007: para. 12.5) attempts to clarify this, stating that section 44:

'only applies if the child's lack of capacity to make a decision for themselves is caused by an impairment or disturbance that affects how their mind or brain works.'

If the lack of capacity is owing to immaturity or some other cause, then the ordinary charge of child cruelty or neglect could be applied.

The assessment of capacity: its contemporary legal origins

The capacity test, as described by Hale & Fortin (2010), can be seen to derive from several key judgments in case law. The first was the well-known case *Re C (refusal of treatment)* [1994], which was heard by Mr Justice Thorpe (as he then was) in the High Court.

In *Re C*, the issue was whether a man detained in Broadmoor high-security psychiatric hospital and who experienced persecutory delusions could make a decision about the treatment of his gangrenous leg. The medical advice was that it should be amputated, but the patient was refusing surgery.

In his judgment, the judge concluded that C had the right of self-determination and said:

'(1)   When considering the capacity that entitled an individual to refuse treatment, the question to be decided was whether it had been established that the patient's capacity was so reduced by his chronic mental illness that he did not understand the nature, purpose and effects of the proposed treatment.

(2)   The decision-making process could be analysed in three stages: (i) comprehending and retaining treatment information; (ii) believing it; and (iii) weighing it in the balance to arrive at a choice.

(3)   Applying that test, the presumption that C had the right of self-determination had not been displaced. Although his general capacity was impaired by schizophrenia, it had not been established that he did not sufficiently understand the nature, purpose and effects of the treatment. He had understood and had arrived at a clear choice.'

Incidentally, the three-pronged test in the second paragraph was derived from Dr Eastman, the forensic psychiatrist involved in the case.

The test was applied in a case heard by Mr Justice Wall (*Re C (Detention: Medical Treatment)* [1997]). This concerned a 16-year-old who could not be detained under the MHA because the establishment she was being treated in was not registered for this purpose. Additionally, owing to the complexities of the case, some kind of court order was needed to legitimise the treatment proposed. Ultimately, she was detained and treated under the *parens patriae* jurisdiction of the court.

The test was then refined by Lord Justice Butler-Sloss in *Re MB (Medical treatment)* [1997], another well-known case that concerns a Caesarian section on a woman with a needle phobia. The judge argued that:

'although it might be thought that irrationality sits uneasily with competence to decide, panic indecisiveness and irrationality in themselves do not as such amount to incompetence, but they may be symptoms or evidence of incompetence',

and

'she was incapable of making a decision at all. She was at that moment suffering an impairment of her mental functioning which disabled her. She was temporarily incompetent. In the emergency the doctors would be free to administer the anaesthetic if that were in her best interests.'

So at this crucial moment this patient did not have capacity and the doctors were acting in her best interests.

How does this help us with an assessment of capacity? In brief, quite a lot of context needs to be taken into account.

The starting point for an assessment of capacity in a young person aged 16 or 17 is just the same as for an adult over 18. The two-stage test of capacity is described in the Code of Practice (Department for Constitutional Affairs, 2007: p. 41):

- '• Does the person have an impairment of the mind or brain, or is there some sort of disturbance affecting the way their mind or brain works? (It does not matter whether this disturbance is temporary or permanent.)
- • If so, does that impairment or disturbance mean that the person is unable to make the decision in question at the time it needs to be made?'

What, then, is meant by an impairment or disturbance of the mind or brain? The Code (on p. 44) gives the following examples:

- '• conditions associated with some forms of mental illness
- • dementia
- • significant learning disabilities
- • the long-term effects of brain damage
- • physical or medical conditions that cause confusion, drowsiness or loss of consciousness
- • delirium
- • concussion following a head injury, and
- • the symptoms of alcohol or drug use.'

In considering the second part of the test, the Code states (at para. 4.13) that the person must be given all the practical help they need to help them make the decision. When it comes to the ability to make a decision, the Code suggests (on p. 45) that a person cannot make a decision if they cannot:

- '1. understand information about the decision to be made (the Act calls this 'relevant information')
- 2. retain that information in their mind
- 3. use or weigh that information as part of the decision-making process, or
- 4. communicate their decision (by talking, using sign language or any other means).'

Each of these aspects will now be considered in detail (see also Brindle *et al*, 2015: pp. 33–35 and Puri *et al*, 2012: pp. 158–159).

► By understanding is meant the degree to which an individual has grasped the information presented. It depends on a number of related cognitive abilities, and the way the information is presented to the person (for example, using visual prompts or appropriate interpreters) is of central importance. Brindle *et al* (p. 34) suggest some useful prompts, including:

  ► What is your understanding of the condition that you have?
  ► What are the benefits (or the risks) of the treatments?

► Retaining may be affected by memory or attention and by anxiety states.

► Using or weighing the information is a subtle task and can give the assessor information on how the person is prioritising different options and considering the consequences of each. What the assessor is attempting to get is an account of how the person has come to the decision they have made of how they explain their reasoning. Clinicians should be alert to the matter of undue influence, especially on this aspect of capacity, which might be due to the dominance of a symptom (such as the desire to lose weight in a young person with anorexia nervosa) or the overbearing influence of, for example, a religious group or an adult over the young person. Possible prompts might include:

  ► Can you tell me how you reached your decision?
  ► What made you decide to choose X rather than Y?

► Communicating the decision may clearly be affected by impairments in language or severe illness. Using whatever form of communication the person prefers, the question should be asked:

  ► Can you tell me what you have decided to do?

In addition to these more general questions, the psychiatrist will also need to examine the young person's mental state. More detailed assessments of cognitive ability may be warranted and may already have been performed as a result of psychological testing (see Brindle *et al*, 2015: pp. 38–40).

In this context it is important to note that the Code of Practice makes a distinction between not having capacity within the meaning of the MCA and just being overwhelmed by the moment (i.e. a psychological response to what is happening – see paragraph 12.13 below). The latter should not be considered to be a demonstration of lack of capacity within the terms of the Act, although clinically this may not always be very obvious.

General points on the assessment of capacity

► A lack of capacity requires proof.

► Assessment might need to be ongoing, as capacity may fluctuate or may vary with different treatments being proposed.

► Greater certainty is needed if the proposed interventions are more serious.

- ► The standard of proof is the balance of probabilities.
- ► The person alleging incapacity should prove it.
- ► There are specific tests concerning capacity to perform certain acts (such as make a will, make a gift, enter a contract, litigate and marry) which the MCA does not replace (Department for Constitutional Affairs, 2007: pp. 51–52).
- ► Capacity may fluctuate.

Application of the MCA to young people aged 16 and 17

As we have seen, the MCA does generally apply to 16- and 17-year-olds if they lack capacity.

What does the Code of Practice say about the application of the Act to this group? The following paragraphs are from the Code (Department for Constitutional Affairs, 2007: pp. 220–223).

'Background information concerning competent young people

12.13 Even where a young person is presumed to have legal capacity to consent to treatment, they may not necessarily be able to make the relevant decision. As with adults, decision-makers should assess the young person's capacity to consent to the proposed care or treatment If a young person lacks capacity to consent within section 2(1) of the Act because of an impairment of, or a disturbance in the functioning of, the mind or brain then the Mental Capacity Act will apply in the same way as it does to those who are 18 and over. If however they are unable to make the decision for some other reason, for example because they are overwhelmed by the implications of the decision, the Act will not apply to them and the legality of any treatment should be assessed under common law principles.

12.14 If a young person has capacity to agree to treatment, their decision to consent must be respected. Difficult issues can arise if a young person has legal and mental capacity and refuses consent – especially if a person with parental responsibility wishes to give consent on the young person's behalf. The Family Division of the High Court can hear cases where there is disagreement. The Court of Protection has no power to settle a dispute about a young person who is said to have the mental capacity to make the specific decision.

12.15 It may be unclear whether a young person lacks capacity within section 2(1) of the Act. In those circumstances, it would be prudent for the person providing care or treatment for the young person to seek a declaration from the court.

If the young person lacks capacity to make care or treatment decisions

12.16 Under the common law, a person with parental responsibility for a young person is generally able to consent to the young person receiving care or medical treatment where they lack capacity under section 2(1) of the Act. They should act in the young person's best interests.

12.17 However if a young person lacks the mental capacity to make a specific care or treatment decision within section 2(1) of the Act, healthcare staff providing treatment, or a person providing care to the young person, can carry out treatment or care with protection from liability (section 5) whether or not a person with parental responsibility consents. They must follow the Act's principles and make sure that the actions they carry out are in the young person's best interests. They must make every effort to work out and consider the young person's wishes, feelings, beliefs and values – both past and present – and consider all other factors in the best interests checklist

12.18 When assessing a young person's best interests, healthcare staff must take into account the views of anyone involved in caring for the young person and anyone interested in their welfare, where it is practical and appropriate to do so. This may include the young person's parents and others with parental responsibility for the young person. Care should be taken not to unlawfully breach the young person's right to confidentiality.

12.19 If a young person has said they do not want their parents to be consulted, it may not be appropriate to involve them (for example, where there have been allegations of abuse).

12.20 If there is a disagreement about whether the proposed care or treatment is in the best interests of a young person, or there is disagreement about whether the young person lacks capacity and there is no other way of resolving the matter, it would be prudent for those in disagreement to seek a declaration or other order from the appropriate court

12.21 There may be particular difficulties where young people with mental health problems require in-patient psychiatric treatment, and are treated informally rather than detained under the Mental Health Act 1983. The Mental Capacity Act and its principles apply to decisions related to the care and treatment of young people who lack mental capacity to consent, including treatment for mental disorder. As with any other form of treatment, somebody assessing a young person's best interests should consult anyone involved in caring for the young person or anyone interested in their welfare, as far as is practical and appropriate. This may include the young person's parents or those with parental responsibility for the young person.'

But the Act does not allow any actions that result in a young person being deprived of their liberty. In such circumstances, detention under the Mental Health Act and the safeguards provided under that Act might be appropriate. Returning to the Code:

'12.22 People may disagree about a young person's capacity to make the specific decision or about their best interests, or it may not be clear whether they lack capacity within section 2(1) or for some other reason. In this situation, legal proceedings may be necessary if there is no other way of settling the disagreement. If those involved in caring for the young person or who are interested in the young person's welfare do not agree with the proposed treatment, it may be necessary for an interested party to make an application to the appropriate court.'

This leaves clinicians with several unanswered questions. How is one to assess whether a young person presenting in a crisis lacks capacity or is just overwhelmed? And what about the implications for admission to an in-patient unit if there is a deprivation of liberty? For young people who do not have capacity, the MHA Code of Practice (Department of Health, 2015: para. 13.53) says:

> 'First, a person who lacks capacity to consent to being accommodated in a hospital for care and/or treatment for mental disorder and who is likely to be deprived of their liberty should never be informally admitted to hospital (whether they are content to be admitted or not).'

Of course, the MHA does provide an alternative framework if certain conditions are met (see Chapter 6). Other than using the MHA, clinicians are currently in a rather uncertain position when it comes to whether or not to seek legal advice (a costly and time-consuming process) in order to apply for a court order. Such an order could be a section 8 order under the Children Act (although this is unlikely for a young person over the age of 16), an order through the Court of Protection, or the inherent jurisdiction of the High Court. The last is an unlimited power to direct any course of action the court sees fit and that might include medical treatment. In each case, clinicians would need to consult the designated administrator of their NHS trust (usually the Mental Health Act administrator), who would seek advice from the organisation's legal team.

To round off the topic, we will now examine the position of the MHA and how these two pieces of legislation occupy their respective places.

Some notes on the relationship between the MHA and the MCA

The first thing to say, with the caveats below, is that it is expedient for the practically minded clinician to consider the MHA first. It should be noted this is not legal advice. Other authors are in agreement with this approach, although they are all primarily considering adults (Puri *et al*, 2012: p. 149; Brindle *et al*, 2015: p. 108; Zigmond & Brindle, 2016: pp. 29–34). Curiously, this approach appeared to have been established in case law in *GJ v The Foundation Trust & Ors* [2009], when the judge said: 'The MHA has primacy'.

However, the same judge seemed to take a somewhat different view in a later case (*AM v South London & Maudsley NHS Foundation Trust* [2013]), which concerned the nature of the interaction between the two legal frameworks. In this case he concluded that:

> 'I agree [...] that my references to the MHA having primacy in *J v Foundation Trust* were made in and should be confined to the application of Case E in that case, and I add that even in that confined context they need some qualification [...] in defined circumstances Parliament has created alternatives that are factors for the relevant decision maker to take into account.'

Use of the MHA will only be relevant in the circumstances defined in Chapter 6, namely that the young person is suffering from a mental disorder of a nature or degree that needs assessment or treatment in hospital, and that hospital admission is necessary for their own safety or that of others, and they are refusing it.

Remember that there are automatic hearings to challenge decisions, rights of appeal and also consent to treatment safeguards, which function to protect the young person's rights under the MHA.

The second thing to say is that the MHA Code of Practice has views about which framework to use (Department of Health, 2015: Chapter 13) and instructs us that the decision to use one legal framework rather than another should not be based on mere preference (para. 13.58). Indeed, there is a discernible encouragement from both the MHA and the MCA Codes to use the MCA rather than the MHA.

However, much of the emphasis in Chapter 13 of the MHA Code is about the choice between using the MCA/DoLS framework as compared with the MHA, and the MCA/DoLS framework does not concern children and young people under the age of 18.

For patients above the age of 16 who have predominantly a physical disorder, the MCA might well be the first choice of legislation (for a succinct paper on using the MCA in the general hospital setting see Humphreys, 2014). However, this must not involve any deprivation of liberty, and restraint of a person who lacks capacity can be used only to prevent harm to that person. Remember too that the threshold for deprivation of liberty has been lowered following the Cheshire West case, namely that a person is deprived of liberty if 'under continuous supervision and control and [...] not free to leave' (see Chapter 1).

It seems likely that the MCA could be useful with 16- and 17-year-olds who lack capacity when either there is no one available with parental responsibility or the person with parental responsibility is not acting in the best interests of the young person. But, again, this will only be the case if the treatment does not involve a deprivation of liberty.

Remember too that if a young person has capacity, within the terms of the MCA, the MCA is not available.

For patients detained on MHA sections 4, 5(2), 5(4), 35, 135 and 136 there is no authority to treat using the powers of the MHA. Therefore, treatment of mental or physical disorders could be given for such people using the MCA if they lacked capacity and refused.

What happens when a person detained under the MHA needs treatment for a physical disorder? This has certainly vexed clinicians (Zigmond & Brindle discuss this in detail in Chapter 3 of their 2016 book). If the physical disorder is a symptom or manifestation of the mental disorder and the patient is subject to a longer-term detention, treatment might be possible using a section 63: see Chapter 6 for more on this. If the physical disorder is unrelated to the mental disorder, then another approach is needed. Two cases have exemplified this recently: *Re AB* [2015] and *An NHS Trust v A* [2015]. The former concerns an adult, but the latter is about a teenage boy whose age is not given.

In *Re AB* the difficulties of how to sanction treatment for a physical disorder (a serious cardiac condition requiring surgery) in an adult patient detained under section 3 of the MHA are considered. The judge first gives thought to whether a further deprivation of liberty could be sanctioned and finds that it is not for someone already detained under the MHA. She then attends to the requirements of Schedule A1 of the MCA, which could be used to authorise a deprivation of liberty so that the treatment can proceed. The conclusion is that it cannot, and the patient's physical treatment is sanctioned by the inherent jurisdiction of the court.

In the case of *An NHS Trust v A*, however, the judge is far less sanguine. In this case a teenage boy with autism detained under section 3 of the MHA needed investigation for the causes of deterioration in his condition. The computerised tomography (CT) scan he was thought to need was going to have to be done under general anaesthetic. Again the issue is whether a detained patient can be eligible to be deprived of his liberty and whether a welfare order can be made by the Court of Protection for the purpose. The judge says:

> 'One might have thought that I would in such circumstances make a simple order declaring that these procedures are in A's best interests and authorising the necessary deprivation of liberty for that purpose, but [in] order to make the necessary declaration of deprivation of liberty, I have to navigate my way [...] through a thicket of legislative drafting which seems to be designed to confuse and which is characterised by extreme opacity. The recent Law Commission report on the reform of this system has highlighted the impenetrability of much of the legislative provisions as one of the most pressing reasons for reform, and the legislative scheme and language here is a veritable smorgasbord of double negatives and subordinate clauses, requiring a navigational exercise from provision to provision, which is an arduous task even for someone who administers justice in this field on a regular basis.'

Ultimately, he concludes that the double negatives have won, the previous judgment in *AB* was mistaken and the boy is eligible to be deprived of his liberty for the purposes of the proposed treatment. He notes that the DoLS Code of Practice (Ministry of Justice, 2008) confirmed that interpretation.

Both of these cases raise, apart from the obvious matter of the complexity of the legislation, the difficulty of transferring detained patients elsewhere for medical investigations and/or treatment. In part, there are limitations on where these interventions can be provided (with certain establishments not being registered to receive detained patients) and also how to authorise a medical intervention when it amounts to a deprivation of liberty if the patient does not or cannot consent. In these circumstances for a young person, a court order would need to be considered.

Conclusion

The MCA is applicable to young people from 16 onwards. However, there are a number of features not relevant for 16- and 17-year-olds, and these include the Deprivation of Liberty Safeguards, which cannot be used for anyone under 18. Clinicians dealing with young people need to know about the principles of this Act, capacity assessments and also the interaction between this Act and the MHA.

Although the MCA has been considered visionary and empowering by the House of Lords (2014), widespread difficulty has been acknowledged over its implementation and the understanding of it by professionals. As a consequence, it has not met the expectations it raised.

The difficulty for clinicians in child mental health is that this Act cannot be used in emergencies (which are the most complex and difficult situations to manage) when a young person's treatment might involve a deprivation of liberty. Further work on the gap in statutory provision for this sort of problem is being undertaken and changes are likely soon.

CHAPTER 8

Juvenile justice

Bowlby's seminal paper on juvenile thieves (Bowlby, 1944) reminds us of the important roots of child psychiatry, which began with the delinquent child. Some 70 years later, the Prison Reform Trust (2016) has published Lord Laming's review into why 61% of 15- to 18-year-old girls and 33% of boys in custody have spent time in care. The review also investigates why, although fewer than 1% of all children in England are in care, looked after children aged between 10 and 17 are five times as likely to be convicted, or subject to a final warning or reprimand, than other children.

Quite apart from ethical and societal considerations, there is a strong economic argument for keeping children and young people out of the so-called secure estate. The number of young people up to the age of 18 held in custody in the secure estate in June 2015 was 986 (Youth Justice Board, 2013a), and the average cost per year for each young person in a secure children's home was £212000, in a secure training centre it was £178000 and in a young offender institution was £60000 (based on 2012–2013 prices; Youth Justice Board, 2013b).

This chapter is not intended to cover ground extensively discussed elsewhere. In particular, there is much written about the forensic services available for children and young people (e.g. Bailey & Delmage, 2010). Report writing is covered in sources such as Richardson & Casswell (2010). This chapter considers more general matters concerning children and young people who may be known to CAMHS and who come into contact with the criminal justice system. Starting with an overview of detention in custody, relevant rights under the European Convention on Human Rights (ECHR) where they apply to youth justice are highlighted. There are some brief notes on secure accommodation and on restraint. The age of criminal responsibility and the very young offender are then discussed, followed by the steps in the process of contact with the criminal justice system, from interviewing with an appropriate adult to participating in a trial and sentencing. Finally, there is a note on the role of the youth offending team and a brief description of the so-called forensic sections of Part III of the MHA.

The CAMHS clinician may come into contact with children and young people involved with the criminal justice system by being the first health professional to assess them before they enter it or by receiving responsibility for continuing psychiatric care once the young person is returned to the community. Certainly, rates of psychiatric disorder in this group of young people are very high: somewhere between 50 and 100%, depending on the study (Bailey & Delmage, 2010). Young people in long-term care and those requiring special education are at particular risk. Many other childhood psychiatric disorders can be associated with offending, including attention-deficit hyperactivity disorder (ADHD), substance misuse, history of sexual and physical abuse, psychosis and intellectual (learning) disability (Bailey & Delmage, 2010).

The overnight detention of young people in custody

The practice of detaining children and young people in custody has apparently been prevalent in the UK. A report published by the Howard League for Penal Reform (2011) analyses 53 000 overnight detentions of children under 16 years of age in England and Wales in 2008 and 2009:

- ▶ 4 were of children under 10 years old, i.e. under the age of criminal responsibility
- ▶ 1674 (3%) were of 10- and 11-year-olds, a group for whom there are legal protections against overnight detention
- ▶ 11 540 (22%) were of children under 14 (the European average age of criminal responsibility)
- ▶ 27 804 (53%) were of 15- and 16-year-olds
- ▶ 10 845 (21%) were of girls
- ▶ 10 050 (19%) were of Black and minority ethnic children (the remainder were White).

These data were obtained from requests under the Freedom of Information Act and it should be noted that only 24 out of a total of 43 police services in England and Wales responded.

The reasons for the detentions included offences, lack of parental availability, lack of other appropriate adults to challenge the detention, and lack of alternative, i.e. local authority, accommodation. The report makes the point that detaining children and young people in police cells is routine, and that England and Wales are outliers compared with the rest of Europe in taking a more punitive approach to children and young people who break the law.

Newbury (2011) notes a 295% rise in the number of 10- to 14-year-olds detained between 1997 and 2007. She understands these figures to represent an increasing use of custody either for minor offending or because other criminal justice measures were failing.

Detentions in a police cell specifically as a result of using section 136 of the Mental Health Act were not mentioned in either of these reports.

As a result of extensive public and professional campaigning and action, it should now be increasingly rare for children and young people to be taken into police custody under section 136. This recent change and how it came about is discussed in more detail in Chapter 6.

What about human rights and UN Conventions?

Clearly, several articles of the Human Rights Act 1998 are relevant when considering children and adolescents and the criminal justice system. In Chapter 2, the case of *T v United Kingdom (Application 24724/94)* [2000] is described, which was found to breach Article 6. One of the two 10-year-old defendants was found not to have received a fair trial. Chapter 2 also mentioned the UN Convention on the Rights of the Child 1989, known also as the UNCRC or the CRC. Although this is not legally enforced in the UK, it was ratified by the UK in 1991.

The UNCRC has several articles that relate to youth justice. The main ones, as highlighted by Howard League for Penal Reform (2008: p. 4), are Articles 3, 37 and 40. The relevant key points of these can be summarised as follows:

▶ Article 3(1): the best interests of the child must be a primary consideration in all actions undertaken by the courts, administrative authorities and legislative bodies

▶ Article 3(2): the government must take appropriate legislative and administrative measures to ensure that children receive the protection and care necessary for their well-being

▶ Article 37(a): juvenile offenders must not be subjected to torture or other cruel, inhuman or degrading treatment or punishment, and no one under 18 years of age must be sentenced to life imprisonment without possibility of release

▶ Article 37(b): children must not be deprived of their liberty unlawfully or arbitrarily. Arrest, detention or imprisonment of a child must be used only as a measure of last resort and for the shortest possible time

▶ Article 40: the justice system should treat children in an age-appropriate manner that promotes their sense of dignity and worth, encourages their respect for the human rights of others and works towards their reintegration to play a constructive role in society.

The three ways in which a child or adolescent with a mental disorder can be lawfully detained are:

▶ as a result of a secure accommodation order using section 25 of the Children Act 1989

▶ as a result of a sentence from a court for a criminal act

▶ under the Mental Heath Act 1983.

Aspects of each of these will be considered below (but only relevant forensic sections under Part III of the MHA: sections under Part II are discussed in Chapter 6).

It should be noted that secure accommodation can refer to any kind of accommodation used for the purpose of restricting liberty, such as locked wards in psychiatric hospitals or secure units. Case law (*R v Northampton Juvenile Court, ex p Hammersmith and Fulham LBC* [1985] FLR 192) has established that it might even include a maternity ward with controlled access when nurses are instructed not to allow a patient to leave (Hale, 2010: p. 96).

Secure accommodation

Although section 25 of the Children Act and various sections of the Mental Health Act can provide authority to deprive a child of their liberty, this is where the similarity between the Children Act and the Mental Health Act ends. It is important to note that the Mental Health Act is used for the compulsory detention and treatment of a person's mental disorder: section 25 of the Children Act does not give any authority to provide medical treatment.

Secure orders can be made by the criminal and family courts (in what were previously known as family proceedings: see Harbour, 2008). They cannot be made for children under the age of 13 without the approval of the Secretary of State. Under section 25 of the Children Act, a local authority can apply for a Secure Accommodation Order for a young person in its care only if certain criteria apply:

▶ the young person has a history of absconding and is likely to abscond from any other type of accommodation, and

▶ if they do abscond they are likely to suffer significant harm, or

▶ if they are kept in any other type of accommodation they are likely to injure themselves or others.

In addition:

▶ approval of the Secretary of State is required for a child under the age of 13

▶ parental agreement is needed if the young person is not on a care order (if parental consent is not given, an interim care order would be needed as well as a secure accommodation order).

In an emergency, a Director's Order (i.e. and order signed by the director of the local authority) can be obtained for up to 72 hours if the criteria are met. A Secure Accommodation Order lasts for 3 months initially, but is renewable for 6 months at a time. If a young person is on remand from a criminal court different rules apply.

Regardless of the duration of the order, if during its course the child no longer meets the criteria, the local authority is obliged to remove the child from secure accommodation (Puri *et al*, 2012: p. 194). Secure accommodation is currently governed by The Children (Secure Accommodation) Regulations 1991 and the reader is referred to these for further detail.

A note on the use of control and restraint

Clinicians should be aware of regulations and guidelines concerning the control and restraint of children and young people admitted to psychiatric settings. Such restrictions on a young person may fall within the 'ordinary acceptable parental restrictions upon the movements of a child', a phrase taken from *Re K (Secure accommodation order: right to liberty)* [2001]. But if they do not, consideration will need to be given to using the Children Act, the Mental Health Act or a court order to authorise these restrictions (Harbour, 2008: p. 58).

▶ The Children's Homes (England) Regulations 2015 (section 20) govern the use of restraint in children's homes.

▶ Youth Justice Board (2011) guidelines concern behaviour management of children and young people in secure accommodation.

▶ The MHA Code of Practice (Department of Health, 2015: Chapter 26) provides detailed guidance on restraint and behavioural management across the age range in psychiatric or social care settings. This includes a sample behaviour support plan, observation protocols and how they should be managed, restrictive interventions and how they should be used, policies for seclusion, physical restraint and rapid tranquillisation. Paragraphs 26.52–26.61 are specific to children and adolescents.

The age of criminal responsibility

The principle that children under the age of 10 cannot be guilty of an offence derives from the Children and Young Persons Act 1933 (see Harbour, 2008). However, it had long been assumed that children up to the age of 14 were incapable of forming criminal intent – a presumption known as *doli incapax* – unless it could be proven otherwise. Offenders under the age of 14 were therefore broadly subject to welfare disposals. Since the abolition of *doli incapax* by the Crime and Disorder Act 1998 many organisations, including the Royal College of Psychiatrists (2006), the Howard League for Penal Reform and the Law Lords, have been concerned about the lack of protection for this age group.

In a survey of comparative youth justice systems across Europe, the Howard League for Penal Reform (2008) describes not only that the age of criminal responsibility differs between countries (Table 8.1), but also that

Table 8.1 Ages of criminal responsibility is some European countries

Country	Age of criminal responsibility, years
England and Wales	10
Scotland	8
Northern Ireland	12
Italy	14
Germany	14
Spain	16 (14 in Catalonia)
France	13 (educational measures imposed from the age of 10)

Adapted from Howard League for Penal Reform, 2008: p. 6.

the courts in different countries deal with children in different ways. This makes comparing standards problematic. In France, for example, where the age of criminal responsibility is 13, children aged 10 can receive community or education orders as a result of appearing before a judge. In Scotland, although the age of criminal responsibility is only 8, the juvenile justice system is widely regarded as welfare oriented rather than punishment oriented.

Notwithstanding the problems of comparison, according to this survey the countries that make up the UK have the lowest ages of criminal responsibility. England and Wales also detain more children than any other country in Western Europe: around 3000 children are detained at any one time and some 10000 children on average pass through the secure estate each year (Howard League for Penal Reform, 2008: p. 7).

What about very young offenders?

As a consequence of the age of criminal responsibility in England and Wales, if a child under the age of 10 breaks the law they cannot be charged with committing a criminal offence. However, they can be given either a local child curfew or a child safety order. Under a local child curfew, the police can ban a child from being in a public place between 21.00h and 06.00h, unless accompanied by an adult. It can last for up to 90 days. If a child breaks its curfew a child safety order can be imposed.

A child safety order places the child under the supervision of a youth offending team (see below). The order normally lasts for up to 3 months, but in some cases it can last for up to 12 months.

If a child doesn't comply with the rules of an order, the court can consider whether they should be taken into care.

A section of the gov.uk website has information about this (HM Government, 2014).

The police interview

Being interviewed after arrest is a formal process that is governed by the Police and Criminal Evidence Act 1984, known as PACE, and Code C of its Codes of Practice (Home Office, 2014). Part 2 of the Criminal Justice and Courts Act 2015 amends PACE so that the term 'arrested juvenile' now extends to young people up to the age of 18 rather than up to the age of 17. This means that the age at which a young person is considered a juvenile for the purposes of PACE is now extended.

As highlighted in an authoritative paper by Ventress *et al* (2008), psychiatrists are called on to give advice about fitness to be interviewed by the police. Fitness to be interviewed is described in Annex G of Code C. Clinicians need to know about appropriate adults, how to assess fitness to be interviewed and be familiar with the range of psychopathology that might interfere with this assessment.

Appropriate adults

Whenever the police detain or interview a child or young person (aged 10 to 18), they must inform an appropriate adult as soon as is practicable and invite them to attend. The appropriate adult's role is to protect the young person's interests. Their responsibilities are recorded in detail on the website of the Youth Justice Board (2014a) and include advising, supporting and assisting the young person, ensuring that they understand their rights and helping with communication.

From the police point of view, the preferred appropriate adult will be either the individual's parent/guardian or social worker. If these people are not available, the local youth offending team (YOT) has an obligation to provide an appropriate adult.

A person may not be an appropriate adult if they are the victim, are involved in the offence, are a witness to it or are employed by the police.

Fitness to be interviewed

Annex G of Code C is concerned with whether or not a detainee is put 'at risk' as a result of the interview. By this is meant whether conducting the interview could significantly harm their physical or mental state, or whether anything they say may be considered unreliable in subsequent court proceedings because of their mental state at the time of interview. Code C states that the following must be considered in determining whether the detainee is fit to be interviewed:

'(a)   how the detainee's physical or mental state might affect their ability to understand the nature and purpose of the interview, to comprehend what is being asked and to appreciate the significance of any answers given and make rational decisions about whether they want to say anything;

(b)   the extent to which the detainee's replies may be affected by their physical or mental condition rather than representing a rational and accurate explanation of their involvement in the offence;

(c)   how the nature of the interview, which could include particularly probing questions, might affect the detainee'

(Home Office, 2014: Annex G, para. 3).

Ventress *et al* (2008) give many examples from case law to illustrate the relationship between evidence obtained by interview, often involving confessions, and mental disorders or vulnerabilities. One of these (*R v Delaney* (1988)) concerned a 17-year-old with a low IQ. The case went to appeal and was successful, as the young man's confession was deemed unreliable. They also list other symptoms that may render a person unfit to be interviewed, including (but not confined to) distractibility, arousal, intoxication and anxiety. Finally, they set out questions that can be used in assessing fitness to be interviewed, which they consider to be a modified capacity test. Thus:

► Can the young person understand:
  ► the questions being put to them?
  ► the nature and significance of the police caution?
  ► the nature and purpose of the interview?
  ► the significance of what is being asked?
  ► the significance of any answers given?
► Can they make reasoned and rational decisions about whether they want to say anything?
► Does their mental state adversely affect their capacity to be accurate or tell the truth?
► Would the interview process result in a significant deterioration in their condition?

Detained with a mental disorder without charge

The particular aspect of the process that can incur difficulty in emergencies is the arrest of a young person with a mental disorder who has, say, assaulted someone but has not been placed on a section 135 or 136 under the MHA (see Chapter 6). As is well known, for most common offences the police may detain a person without charge for a maximum of 24 hours. If a charge is not made because an interview cannot be properly carried out then the person must be released. The police will usually be keen to keep to this time limit, although Code C allows for an extension to be made of 12 hours; further extensions can be made only by a magistrates' court (Home Office 2014: para. 15). A bed may be needed urgently if hospital treatment is thought necessary and the CAMHS clinician will find themselves under a great deal of pressure to relocate the young person quickly.

A fair trial?

Requirements for a fair trial are stipulated in Article 6 of the ECHR. In the case of *T v United Kingdom (Application 24724/94)* [2000], which is discussed in Chapter 2, Article 6 was found to have been breached even though some special arrangements had been made for the trial of the child defendants.

Practice directions have subsequently been issued and the Crown Prosecution Service (2015*a*), in its guidance on youths with mental disorders including learning disability, has set out requirements for trial procedure. These include that:

'• The youth has to understand what he is said to have done wrong
  • The court must be satisfied that the youth had the means of knowing that an act or omission was wrong at the time of the act or omission
  • The youth had to understand what, if any, defences were available to him
  • The youth must have a reasonable opportunity to make relevant representations if he wished to do so
  • The youth must have the opportunity to consider what representations he wished to make once he had understood the issues involved.'

Furthermore, the youth court should take appropriate steps to enable a youth with a learning disability or mental impairment to participate in the trial. These steps include:

'• Keeping the youth's cognitive functioning in mind
  • Using concise and simple language
  • Having regular breaks
  • Taking additional time to explain court proceedings
  • Being proactive in ensuring the youth has access to support
  • Explaining and ensuring the claimant understands the ingredients of the charge
  • Explaining the possible outcomes and sentences
  • Ensuring cross examination is carefully controlled so that questions are short and clear and frustration is minimised.'

If it becomes apparent during the course of the hearing that the person is unable to participate effectively, the judge can halt the proceedings.

Fitness to plead and stand trial

Fitness to plead in the Crown Court follows a formula first articulated in 1836 known as the Prichard criteria, but reiterated in the case of *John (M)* [2003]. They are whether a defendant can understand the charges, decide whether to plead guilty or not, challenge a juror, instruct a representative, follow the course of proceedings and give evidence in his or her own defence (Bevan, 2014).

While fitness to stand trial is governed by this process in the Crown Court, there is no equivalent test of this in magistrates' or youth courts.

The Crown Prosecution Service (2015b) states that only in exceptional circumstances should the youth court exercise its power to halt proceedings before hearing evidence on the substantive issue of the case. It emphasises that it is for the court, not the doctors, to decide whether a trial should take place. Furthermore, if the court decides not to proceed with a criminal trial because the youth cannot take an effective part in the proceedings, it should consider whether to undertake a trial of the facts. It recommends that:

> 'Proceedings should be stayed as an abuse of process before the fact finding exercise only if there would be no useful purpose served by making a finding on the facts. The fact that the youth does not or cannot take any part in the proceedings does not render them unfair or in any way improper' (Crown Prosecution Service, 2015a).

This seems likely to be the subject of further review by the Law Commission.

Sentencing

The section on youth offenders on the Crown Prosecution Service website has updated guidance on young people and the criminal justice system in England and Wales and the reader is referred to this for detailed information (Crown Prosecution Service, 2015c). Reprimands and warnings for the under-18s were effectively abolished in 2013 and youth cautions and youth conditional cautions have replaced them (Crown Prosecution Service, 2015d). These are formal out-of-court disposals.

Once in court, the Criminal Justice and Immigration Act 2008 simplifies the range of youth sentences now available. The principal sentences for offences committed on or after 30 November 2009 are:

► referral order
► youth rehabilitation order
► detention and training order

(Crown Prosecution Service, 2015d).

Note that a youth rehabilitation order can have a mental health treatment requirement attached to it provided that:

► the young person will comply with it, and
► the condition is susceptible to treatment but does not require a hospital order or guardianship order (see below);
► arrangements can be specified in the order, including where the treatment is to occur

(see also Puri et al, 2012).

In addition, sentences such as compensation orders, fines, reparation orders, hospital and guardianship orders continue to be available.

The Crown Court also retains a number of sentencing powers for serious crimes (Crown Prosecution Service, 2015*d*).

Youth offending teams

These multidisciplinary teams were established by the Crime and Disorder Act 1998. A youth offending team (YOT) works with other agencies, such as the police, probation, health, children's and education services, and coordinates the youth justice services in a local area. The YOT works with children and young people who have come into contact with the police or have been given a criminal justice disposal.

To undertake this work, offending-related risks and needs are assessed by the YOT practitioner. The findings of this assessment are used to develop an intervention plan.

In a large study of a cohort of more than 13 000 children and young people seen by 30 YOTs in England and Wales, Wilson (2013) studied these plans and found that (controlling for offender characteristics) the greater the number of face-to-face contacts between the young person and their YOT worker, the less likely they were to reoffend over a 1 year period. Whether or not the Youth Justice Board has been influenced by this and similar studies, it now provides considerable online resources for the assessment of young offenders (Youth Justice Board, 2014*b*). These address reoffending risks and provide practitioners with detailed guidance about court work, risk assessment and the eligibility for multi-agency public protection arrangements (MAPPA).

Youth detention accommodation

Following the Legal Aid, Sentencing and Punishment of Offenders Act 2012 (the LASPO Act) all children and young people up to the age of 18 remanded by a court in criminal proceedings will now be 'looked after' (enter the care of the local authority). This Act, in sections 91–107 and Schedule 12, also describes a number of changes to the youth remand framework, as summarised in a circular from the Ministry of Justice (2012):

'•   10 to 17 year olds are treated according to the same remand framework and conditions for custodial remand regardless of their age and gender;

•   the court must first consider whether to remand a child on bail. Where the court refuses bail it should then consider whether to remand to local authority accommodation or whether, if the child is aged 12–17, the conditions for a remand to youth detention accommodation are met;

•   17 year olds who are remanded will be treated in the same way as younger children. They may therefore now be remanded to local authority accommodation;

•   a 12–17 year old can be remanded to youth detention accommodation if they meet one of two sets of conditions; the first are based on the type of offending and the second are based on the history of absconding or offending together with whether there is a real prospect of a custodial sentence; and

- every child remanded to youth detention accommodation will now be treated as "looked after" by their designated local authority.'

Youth detention accommodation (YDA) is defined in the LASPO Act and currently comprises a secure children's home, secure training centre or young offender institution (YOI). Specific criteria must be met in order to place a child in one of these settings and the type of offence and the history taken into account.

Secure children's homes in England are run by local authorities in conjunction with the Department for Education in England. There is one secure children's home in Wales. They generally accommodate remanded or sentenced children aged 12 to 14 and 'at-risk' girls and boys up to the age of 16. Secure training centres, of which there are three in England, offer secure provision to sentenced or remanded young people aged 12–17. Young offender institutions can accommodate young offenders aged between 15 and 21. These institutions tend to be larger than secure children's homes and secure training centres, with lower ratios of staff to young people (Ministry of Justice, 2015b).

Further guidance on the placement of children and young people who are in the care system and arrested, charged or on remand can be found in documents issued by the Department for Education (2015) and the Ministry of Justice (2012).

The forensic sections of the Mental Health Act

Detention under the Mental Health Act using the civil section 2 or 3 (described in Part II of the Act) can, of course, be used for the assessment and/or treatment of a young person with a mental disorder. Part III of the Act, however, specifically deals with mentally disordered offenders and lists the so-called forensic sections.

It is possible for a patient to be detained on both a civil and a forensic section at the same time.

The range of hospital orders available for children and young people is the same as that for adults. As they are not in common use, only notes on the differing kinds are given here and in Table 8.2. The reader is referred to Richards & Moghul (2010) and the South London and Maudsley Foundation Trust (2013) for complete descriptions.

Detention of young offenders before sentencing

- ▶ **Section 35** For assessment of mental disorder in an accused person remanded to hospital by a Crown Court or youth court. Medical treatment cannot be given without consent. A section 12 doctor is needed to give evidence to the court. A section 35 lasts for 28 days, but is renewable.

Table 8.2 Summary of key information governing the detention of patients under Part III of the Mental Health Act

	Section 35	Section 36	Sections 37/41	Section 38	Sections 47/49	Sections 48/49
By whom?	One registered medical practitioner	Two registered medical practitioners (one section 12 approved)	Two registered medical practitioners (one section 12 approved)	Two registered medical practitioners (one section 12 approved), one employed by the admitting hospital	Two registered medical practitioners (one section 12 approved)	Two registered medical practitioners (one section 12 approved)
Can the responsible clinician move the patient?	Responsible clinician cannot move, send on leave or discharge	Responsible clinician cannot move, send on leave or discharge	Responsible clinician cannot move, send on leave or discharge (if the patient is restricted)	Responsible clinician cannot move, send on leave or discharge	Responsible clinician cannot move, send on leave or discharge	Responsible clinician cannot move, send on leave or discharge
Can medical treatment be given using the authority of the MHA Part IV?	Cannot give medical treatment for mental disorder without the patient's consent	Can give medication under Part IV	Can give medication under Part IV	Can give medication under Part IV	Can give medication under Part IV	Can give medication under Part IV
How long does the section last?	28 days, renewable up to 12 weeks	28 days, renewable up to 12 weeks	Until discharged by Secretary of State/tribunal/responsible clinician	12 weeks, renewable up to 12 months	Until the end of the sentence. Patient remains detained but without restriction	Depends on the outcome of the legal case
Where next for the patient?	Return to court	Return to court	Can be conditionally or absolutely discharged or placed on a CTO	Return to court	Return to prison	Return to prison

Note: Patients detained under Part III treatment orders have the same entitlement to aftercare under section 117 as Part II detained patients. Reproduced with permission from Zigmond & Brindle, 2016: p. 67.

▶ **Section 36** For assessment and treatment of mental disorder in an accused person remanded to hospital by a Crown Court. Treatment can be given without consent, if necessary. Two doctors are needed, one of whom must be section 12 approved. A section 36 lasts for 28 days but is renewable.

▶ **Section 36**, and **sections 37, 47** and **48** (below) stipulate requirements concerning the definition of mental disorder similar to those in the sections in Part II of the Act (see Chapter 6). That is to say, it is of a nature or degree making it appropriate for detention in hospital, and appropriate medical treatment is available.

▶ **Section 48** For assessment and treatment of mental disorder in a remanded person awaiting trial. Section 48 is rarely used and is invariably given with a section 49 (see below). Treatment can be given without consent, if necessary. Two doctors are needed, one of whom must be section 12 approved.

Detention of young offenders after sentencing

▶ **Section 37** (hospital order) For hospital treatment with or without section 41. If without a 41 (see below) the person can be discharged by the responsible clinician at any time (rather like a section 3). The section allows for treatment to be given without consent, if necessary. Two doctors are needed, one of whom must be section 12 approved. A section 37 can last for up to 6 months.

▶ **Section 38** For children and young people who have been convicted, to allow further assessment when it is unclear whether they should be sentenced to hospital or prison. The section allows for treatment without consent. Two doctors are needed, one of whom must be section 12 approved. Initially for a period of 12 weeks, it can be renewed for up to 12 months.

▶ **Section 41** (restriction order) When the grounds for a section 37 are met, this order can be attached to a young person over the age of 14 to prevent the responsible clinician from moving, sending on leave or discharging the young person without the permission of the Secretary of State for the Ministry of Justice.

▶ **Section 45A** (limitation direction) For serious offences and immediate admission to psychiatric hospital. This is an infrequently used so-called hybrid order, intended to ensure that convicted offenders who could normally attract a significant custodial sentence do not end up serving significantly less time in the secure psychiatric system. Equally, they are not denied access to necessary treatment for their mental disorder. Once a mental disorder is improved, the remaining sentence may be served in prison.

▶ **Section 47** (transfer direction) For the hospital treatment of a convicted and imprisoned person. Treatment can be given without consent if necessary. Two doctors are needed, one of whom must be section 12 approved. Invariably given with a section 49, this can be made for 6 months initially.

▶ **Section 49** (restriction direction) Invariably used with section 47 or 48, which ensures that the court (for those on remand) or the Ministry of Justice (for sentenced prisoners) are in charge of discharge rather than the responsible clinician.

Conclusion

The CAMHS clinician may come into contact with children and young people about to enter the criminal justice system or receive responsibility for continuing psychiatric care once a young person is returned to the community.

Many children in custody have spent time in care. This chapter is therefore relevant for all CAMHS clinicians, in giving an overview of the detention of young people in custody. Human Rights Act/ECHR rights where they apply to youth justice are highlighted and there are some brief notes on secure accommodation and on restraint. It is useful for clinicians to know the steps in the process from first contact between a young person and the criminal justice system, through to interviewing with an appropriate adult present and then to participating in a trial and sentencing. They should also be aware of the role of the youth offending team and the so-called forensic sections of Part III of the MHA.

References

Bailey, S. & Delmage, E. (2010) Forensic services. In *Child and Adolescent Mental Health Services: An Operational Handbook* (2nd edn) (eds G. Richardson, I. Partridge & J. Barrett): pp. 284–292. RCPsych Publications.

Barber, P., Brown, R. & Martin, D. (2012) *Mental Health Law in England and Wales: A Guide for Mental Health Professionals* (2nd edn). Sage.

Bevan, E. (2014) Unfit to plead in the Magistrates' and Youth Courts? *Criminal Law and Justice Weekly*, **178**(23), 6 June.

Black, D., Harris-Hendriks, J. & Wolkind, S. (1998) *Child Psychiatry and the Law* (3rd edn). Royal College of Psychiatrists.

Bowlby, J. (1944) Forty-four juvenile thieves: their characters and home-life. *International Journal of Psycho-Analysis*, **25**, 19–53.

Brindle, N., Branton, T, Stansfield, A., *et al* (2015) *A Clinician's Brief Guide to the Mental Capacity Act* (2nd edn). RCPsych Publications.

British Medical Association (2010) *Children and Young People Toolkit*. BMA.

Care Quality Commission (2010) *Monitoring the Use of the Mental Health Act in 2009/10*. CQC.

Care Quality Commission (2014) *Monitoring the Mental Health Act in 2012/13*. CQC.

Care Quality Commission (2015) *Monitoring the Mental Health Act in 2013/4*. CQC.

Courts and Tribunals Judiciary (2012) *The Structure of the Courts*. Courts and Tribunals Judiciary (https://www.judiciary.gov.uk/wp-content/uploads/2012/08/courts-structure-0715.pdf). Accessed 29 July 2016.

Crown Prosecution Service (2015a) *Trial Procedure for Youths with Mental Disorders Including Learning Disabilities*. CPS (http://www.cps.gov.uk/legal/v_to_z/youth_offenders/#a19). Accessed 29 July 2016.

Crown Prosecution Service (2015b) *Principles Guiding the Decision to Prosecute*. CPS (http://www.cps.gov.uk/legal/v_to_z/youth_offenders/#a09). Accessed 29 July 2016.

Crown Prosecution Service (2015c) *Youths with Mental Disorders, including Learning Disabilities*. CPS (http://www.cps.gov.uk/legal/v_to_z/youth_offenders/#a17). Accessed 29 July 2016.

Crown Prosecution Service (2015d) *Sentencing*. CPS (http://www.cps.gov.uk/legal/v_to_z/youth_offenders/#a37). Accessed 29 July 2016.

Curtice, M. & James, L. (2016) Faith, ethics and Section 63 of the Mental Health Act 1983. *BJPsych Bulletin*, **40**, 77–81.

Department for Constitutional Affairs (2006) *A Guide to the Human Rights Act 1998: Third Edition*. DCA.

Department for Constitutional Affairs (2007) *The Mental Capacity Act 2005: Code of Practice*. TSO (The Stationery Office).

Department for Education (2015) *The Children Act 1989 Guidance and Regulations. Volume 2: Care Planning, Placement and Case Review*. Department for Education.

Department of Health (2003) *Confidentiality: NHS Code of Practice*. Department of Health.

Department of Health (2004) *Best Practice Guidance for Doctors and Other Health Professionals on the Provision of Advice and Treatment to Young People under 16 on Contraception, Sexual and Reproductive Health*. Department of Health.

Department of Health (2008) *Mental Health Act 1983: Code of Practice*. TSO (The Stationery Office).

Department of Health (2009) *Reference Guide to Consent for Examination or Treatment* (2nd edn). Department of Health.

Department of Health (2015) *Mental Health Act 1983: Code of Practice*. TSO (The Stationery Office).

Department of Health (2016) *Mental Health Act: Instructions with Respect to the Exercise of an Approval Function in Relation to Approved Clinicians 2015*. Department of Health.

Department of Health & Home Office (2014) *Review of the Operation of Sections 135 and 136 of the Mental Health Act 1983: Report Summary and Recommendations*. Department of Health & Home Office.

Edozien, L. (2015) UK law on consent finally embraces the prudent patient standard. *BMJ*, **350**, h287.7

Faculty of Child and Adolescent Psychiatry (2015) *Survey of In-Patient Admissions for Children and Young People with Mental Health Problems (Faculty Report FR/CAP/01)*. Royal College of Psychiatrists.

Fellow-Smith, E., Hindley, P. & Hughes, N. (2016) *Defining a Health-Based Place of Safety (S136) and Crisis Assessment Sites for Young People under 18* (Position Statement PS02/16). Royal College of Psychiatrists.

Fortin, J. (2014) Children's rights – flattering to deceive? *Child and Family Law Quarterly*, **26**(1), 51–63.

General Medical Council (2007) *0–18 Years: Guidance for All Doctors*. GMC.

General Medical Council (2008) *Consent: Patients and Doctors Making Decisions Together*. GMC.

General Medical Council (2009) *Confidentiality*. GMC.

Gilbar, R. (2012) Medical confidentiality and communication with the patient's family: legal and practical perspectives. *Child and Family Law Quarterly*, **24**, 199–222.

Gilmore, S. & Herring, J. (2011) "No" is the hardest word: consent and children's autonomy. *Child and Family Law Quarterly*, **23**(1), 3–25.

Hale, B. (2010) *Mental Health Law* (5th edn). Sweet & Maxwell.

Hale, B. & Fortin, J. (2010) Legal issues in the care and treatment of children with mental health problems. In *Rutter's Child and Adolescent Psychiatry* (5th edn) (eds M. Rutter, D. Bishop, D. Pine, *et al*), pp. 95–110. Wiley-Blackwell.

Harbour, A. (2008) *Children with Mental Disorder and the Law: A Guide to Law and Practice*. Jessica Kingsley.

Health and Social Care Information Centre (2014) *Inpatients Formally Detained in Hospitals under the Mental Health Act 1983 and Patients Subject to Supervised Community Treatment, England – 2013–2014, Annual Figures*. HSCIC.

Health Research Authority (2015) *What is section 251?* Health Research Authority (http://www.hra.nhs.uk/about-the-hra/our-committees/section-251/what-is-section-251). Accessed 29 July 2016.

Health Select Committee (2013) *Post-Legislative Scrutiny of the Mental Health Act 2007: First Report of Session 2013–14* (HC 584). House of Commons.

Health Select Committee (2014) *Health Committee – Third Report : Children's and Adolescents' Mental Health and CAMHS* (HC342). House of Commons.

Hirst, M. (2015) The expert witness and the criminal courts. Commentary on: When is an expert not an expert? *BJPsych Advances*, **21**, 304–306.

HM Government (2014) *What happens if a child under 10 breaks the law?* (https://www.gov.uk/child-under-10-breaks-law). Accessed 29 July 2016.

HM Government (2015a) *Working Together to Safeguard Children: A Guide to Interagency Working to Safeguard and Promote the Welfare of Children*. TSO (The Stationery Office).

HM Government (2015b) *Information Sharing: Advice for Practitioners Providing Safeguarding Services to Children, Young People, Parents and Carers*. TSO (The Stationery Office).

HM Treasury (2003) *Every Child Matters (Cm 5860)*. TSO (The Stationery Office).

Home Office (2014) *Revised Code of Practice for the Detention, Treatment and Questioning of Persons by Police Officers: Police and Criminal Evidence Act 1984 (PACE) – Code C*. Home Office.

House of Lords (2014) *Mental Capacity Act 2005: Post-Legislative Scrutiny. Select Committee on the Mental Capacity Act 2005: Report of Session 2013–14* (HL Paper 139). TSO (The Stationery Office).

Howard League for Penal Reform (2008) *Punishing Children: A Survey of Criminal Responsibility and Approaches across Europe*. Howard League for Penal Reform.

Howard League for Penal Reform (2011) *Overnight Detention of Children in Police Cells: Summary*. Howard League for Penal Reform.

Humphreys, R. (2014) When and how to treat patients who refuse treatment. *BMJ*, **348**, g2043.

Jackson, E. (2013) *Medical Law: Text, Cases and Materials* (3rd edn). Oxford University Press.

Jones, R. (2014) *Mental Capacity Act Manual*. Sweet & Maxwell.

Kennedy, I. & Grubb, A. (2000) *Medical Law* (3rd edn). Butterworths.

Law Commission (2015) *Mental Capacity and Deprivation of Liberty: A Consultation Paper (Consultation Paper No 222)*. Law Commission.

Law Society (2015a) *Family law changes: information from the Ministry of Justice*. Law Society (https://www.lawsociety.org.uk/support-services/family-court-resources/family-law-changes-information-from-the-ministry-of-justice. Accessed 29 July 2016.

Law Society (2015b) Under 18s. In *Identifying a Deprivation of Liberty: A Practical Guide*. Law Society (https://www.lawsociety.org.uk/support-services/advice/articles/deprivation-of-liberty/Chapter 9). Accessed 29 July 2016.

Maden, T. & Spencer-Lane, T. (2010) *Essential Mental Health Law: A Guide to the Revised MHA and the MCA*. Hammersmith Press.

Martin, J. (2005) *The English Legal System* (4th edn). Hodder Arnold.

Ministry of Justice (2008) *Mental Capacity Act 2005: Deprivation of Liberty Safeguards – Code of Practice to Supplement the Main Mental Capacity Act 2005 Code of Practice*. Ministry of Justice.

Ministry of Justice (2012) *Legal Aid, Sentencing and Punishment of Offenders Act 2012: The New Youth Remand Framework and Amendments to Adult Remand Provisions* (Circular No. 2012/06). Ministry of Justice.

Ministry of Justice (2015a) *Family Court Statistics Quarterly: January to March 2015*. Ministry of Justice.

Ministry of Justice (2015b) *Youth Custody Report: August 2015*. Ministry of Justice.

Ministry of Justice & Department for Education (2014) *A Brighter Future for Family Justice: A Round Up of What's Happened Since the Family Justice Review*. Ministry of Justice, Department for Education.

National Institute for Mental Health in England (2008) *Mental Health Act 2007: New Roles. Guidance for Approving Authorities and Employers on Approved Mental Health Practitioners and Approved Clinicians*. NIMHE.

National Institute for Mental Health in England (2009) *The Legal Aspects of the Care and Treatment of Children and Young People with Mental Disorder: A Guide for Professionals*. Department of Health/NIMHE.

Newbury (2011) Very young offenders and the criminal justice system: are we asking the right questions? *Child and Family Law Quarterly*, **23**(1), 94–114.

Patil, P., Mezey, G. C. & White, S (2013) Characteristics of adolescents placed under section 136 Mental Health Act 1983. *Journal of Forensic Psychiatry and Psychology*, **24**, 610–620.

Penny, C. & Exworthy, T. (2015) A gilded cage is still a cage: Cheshire West widens 'deprivation of liberty'. *British Journal of Psychiatry*, **206**, 91–92.

Prison Reform Trust (2016) *Keeping children in care out of trouble: an independent review*. Prison Reform Trust (http://www.prisonreformtrust.org.uk/ProjectsResearch/CareReview). Accessed 29 July 2016.

Pugh, K. (2008) Getting ready for change. *Mental Health Today*, July/August, 29–31.

Puri, B., Brown, R., McKee, H *et al* (2012) *Mental Health Law: A Practical Guide* (2nd edn). Hodder Arnold.

Richards, S. & Moghul, A. (2010) *Working with the Mental Health Act* (3rd edn). Matrix Training Associates.

Richardson, G. & Casswell, G. (2010) Court work. In *Child and Adolescent Mental Health Services: An Operational Handbook* (2nd edn) (eds G. Richardson, I. Partridge & J. Barrett), pp. 248–258. RCPsych Publications.

Rix, K. J. B. (2011) *Expert Psychiatric Evidence*. RCPsych Publications.

Roch-Bery, C. (2003) What is a Caldicott guardian? *Postgraduate Medical Journal*, **79**, 516–518.

Royal College of Psychiatrists (2006) *Child Defendants* (Occasional Paper OP56). Royal College of Psychiatrists.

Royal College of Psychiatrists (2011) *Standards on the Use of Section 136 of the Mental Health Act 1983 (England and Wales)* (College Report CR159). Royal College of Psychiatrists.

Royal College of Psychiatrists (2013) *Guidance for Commissioners: Service Provision for Section 136 of the Mental Health Act 1983* (Position Statement PS2/2013). Royal College of Psychiatrists.

South London and Maudsley Foundation Trust (2013) *The Maze: A Practical Guide to the Mental Health Act 1983 (Amended 2007)*. South London and Maudsley Foundation Trust.

Thomas, V., Chipchase B, Rippon L, *et al* (2015) The application of mental health legislation in younger children. *BJPsych Bulletin*, **39**, 302–304.

UNICEF (2016) *What is the UNCRC?* UNICEF (http://www.unicef.org.uk/UNICEFs-Work/UN-Convention). Accessed 29 July 2016.

Ventress, M.A., Rix, K.J.B. & Kent, J.H. (2008) Keeping PACE: fitness to be interviewed by the police. *Advances in Psychiatric Treatment*, **14**, 369–381.

Welsh Assembly Government (2008) *Mental Health Act 1983: Code of Practice for Wales*. TSO (The Stationery Office).

Wheeler, R. (2006) Gillick or Fraser? A plea for consistency over competence in children *BMJ*, **332**, 807.

White, R., Harbour, A. & Williams, R. (2004) *Safeguards for Young Minds: Young People and Protective Legislation* (2nd edn). Gaskell.

Wilson, E. (2013) *Youth Justice Interventions – Findings from the Juvenile Cohort Study (JCS)*. Ministry of Justice.

Youth Justice Board (2011) *Behaviour Management across the Secure Estate for Children and Young People: A Study Conducted by Ipsos MORI for the Youth Justice Board*. Youth Justice Board for England and Wales.

Youth Justice Board (2013a) *Youth Custody Report – June 2015: England and Wales*. YJB (https://www.gov.uk/government/publications/youth-custody-data). Accessed 31 August 2015.

Youth Justice Board (2013b) *Children and Young People's Estate Average Sector Prices for 2012–13. Price/Note Information for External and Public Use*. Youth Justice Board for England and Wales.

Youth Justice Board (2014a) *Appropriate adults: guide for youth justice professionals*. gov. uk (https://www.gov.uk/guidance/appropriate-adults-guide-for-youth-justice-professionals). Accessed 29 July 2016.

Youth Justice Board for England and Wales (2014b) *Assess young offenders: case management guidance*. gov.uk (https://www.gov.uk/government/publications/assess-young-offenders). Accessed 29 July 2016.

Zigmund, T. & Brindle, N. (2016) *A Clinician's Brief Guide to the Mental Health Act* (4th edn). RCPsych Publications.

Index

Compiled by Linda English